REFLECTIVE PRACTICE IN NURSING

The Growth of the Professional Practitioner

Other Books of Interest

MENTORING AND PRECEPTORSHIP
A Guide to Support Roles in Clinical Practice
Alison Morton-Cooper and Anne Palmer
0–632–03596–X

EXPANDING THE ROLE OF THE NURSE
The Scope of Professional Practice
Edited by Geoffrey Hunt and Paul Wainright
0–632–03604–4

REFLECTIVE PRACTICE IN NURSING

The Growth of the Professional Practitioner

Editors

ANTHONY M. PALMER

BSc (Hons), RGN, DPSN, PGCEA
Lecturer-Practitioner, Abingdon Community Hospital
and Oxford Brookes University
Editor: Journal of Nursing Management

SARAH BURNS

BA, RGN, SCM, DN (Lond)
Lecturer-Practitioner, John Radcliffe Hospital
and Oxford Brookes University

CHRIS BULMAN

BSc (Hons), MSc, RGN, PGCEA
Lecturer-Practitioner, John Radcliffe Hospital
and Oxford Brookes University

OXFORD

BLACKWELL SCIENTIFIC PUBLICATIONS

LONDON EDINBURGH BOSTON

MELBOURNE PARIS BERLIN VIENNA

© Anthony M. Palmer, Sarah Burns and Chris Bulman 1994

Blackwell Scientific Publications
Editorial Offices:
Osney Mead, Oxford OX2 0EL
25 John Street, London WC1N 2BL
23 Ainslie Place, Edinburgh EH3 6AJ
238 Main Street, Cambridge,
   Massachusetts 02142, USA
54 University Street, Carlton,
   Victoria 3053, Australia

Other Editorial Offices:
Librairie Arnette SA
2, rue Casimir-Delavigne
75006 Paris
France

Blackwell Wissenschafts-Verlag GmbH
Düsseldorfer Str. 38
D-10707 Berlin
Germany

Blackwell MZV
Feldgasse 13
A-1238 Wien
Austria

First published 1994

Set by DP Photosetting, Aylesbury, Bucks
Printed and bound in Great Britain by
Hartnolls Ltd, Bodmin, Cornwall

DISTRIBUTORS
Marston Book Services Ltd
PO Box 87
Oxford OX2 0DT
(*Orders*: Tel: 0865 791155
        Fax: 0865 791927
        Telex: 837515)

USA
Blackwell Scientific Publications, Inc.
238 Main Street
Cambridge, MA 02142
(*Orders*: Tel: 800 759-6102
          617 876-7000)

Canada
Times Mirror Professional Publishing,
Ltd
130 Flaska Drive
Markham, Ontario L6G 1B8
(*Orders*: Tel: 800 268-4178)
          416 470-6739)

Australia
Blackwell Scientific Publications Pty Ltd
54 University Street,
Carlton, Victoria 3053
(*Orders*: Tel: 03 347-5552)

British Library
Cataloguing in Publication Data

A Catalogue record for this book is
available from the British Library

ISBN 0–632–03597–8

Library of Congress
Cataloging in Publication Data
Reflective practice in nursing : the growth
    of the professional practitioner / editors,
    Anthony M. Palmer, Sarah Burns, Chris
    Bulman.
        p.   cm.
    Includes bibliographical references
    and index.
        ISBN 0–632–03597–8
        1. Nursing—Study and teaching.
    2. Nursing—Philosophy.   3. Self-
    evaluation.   4. Self-knowledge,
    Theory of.   I. Palmer, Anthony M.
    II. Burns, Sarah, DN.   III. Bulman, Chris.
        [DNLM: 1. Nursing.   2. Education,
    Nursing.   3. Philosophy, Nursing.
    WY 16R332   1994]
    RT73.R346   1994
    610.73'01—dc 20
    DNLM/DLC
    for Library of Congress   93-38307
                                             CIP

*This book is dedicated
to all students
past and present*

Contents

List of Contributors

Sue Atkins, *MSc, RGN, Dip N, Dip N Ed*, Senior Lecturer, School of Health Care Studies, Oxford Brookes University, Oxford.

Chris Bulman, *BSc (Hons), MSc, RGN, PGCEA*, Lecturer-Practitioner, John Radcliffe Hospital and Oxford Brookes University, Oxford.

Sarah Burns, *BA, RGN, SCM, DN (Lond)*, Lecturer-Practitioner, John Radcliffe Hospital and Oxford Brookes University, Oxford.

Gina Copp, *RGN, Dip N (Lond), Cert Ed, RCNT, M Nurs*, Lecturer Practitioner in Palliative Nursing, School of Health Care Studies, Oxford Brookes University and Sir Michael Sobell House, Churchill Hospital, Oxford.

Sue Duke, *BSc (Hons), RGN ONC*, Lecturer-Practitioner, School of Health Care Studies, Oxford Brookes University and Sir Michael Sobell House, Churchill Hospital, Oxford.

Mary FitzGerald, *RN, DN, Cert Ed (FE), MN*, Postgraduate Student, University of New England, Australia.

Debi Holm, *BA (Hons), RN (A)*, Staff Nurse, Radcliffe Infirmary, Oxford.

Christopher Johns, *RGN, RMN, Cert Ed, MN*, Reader in Advanced Nursing Practice, University of Luton, Luton.

Yvonne M. L'Aguille, *BSc, RGN, FETC*, Senior Sister/Lecturer-Practitioner, Vascular Unit, John Radcliffe Hospital, Oxford.

Kathy Murphy, *SRN, BA (Hons), Dip N, Dip N Ed, MSc*, Senior Lecturer, School of Health Care Studies, Oxford Brookes University, Oxford.

Anthony M. Palmer, *BSc (Hons), RGN, DPSN, PGCEA*, Lecturer-Practitioner, Abingdon Community Hospital and Oxford Brookes University, Oxford.

Brigid Reid, *RGN, BN (Hons), Cert Ed (FE)*, Project Worker, Nursing Development Unit, Bicester Community Hospital, Oxon.

Sarah Stephenson, *BA (Hons), RN*, Staff Nurse, John Radcliffe Hospital, Oxford.

Foreword

Lynne Batehup, *BSc, MSc, DipN, RGN*
Nightingale Institute, Division of Nursing,
King's College, University of London

The context in which nurses practice increasingly reflects instability and constant change as the norm. The health care scene may be driven by any number of competing and conflicting pressures and idealogies, which range from the effects of unrestrained or partially managed market forces, through to government-led social and health care measures to improve health outcomes. Within all this is the drive for cost containment and value for money. Changes in lifestyles and social forces are asserting demands on health and social services which are causing significant strain on the system and those working within it.

There is nothing new about most of this, however, there is acknowledgement that constant change is now a permanent feature of health care delivery, and, with this in mind, major changes in attitudes and practices are required in order to work effectively and to maintain growth and development.

Nurses, as with other disciplines, are expected to be able to respond with flexibility, as well as be proactive and innovative practitioners. The challenge for nurse education is to provide a learning experience that facilitates the so-called 'knowledgeable doer'. My own personal challenge is to propagate the centrality of practice within the setting of higher education so that the basis of our teaching will be rigorous in its approach to enquiry; it should also be research based and critically analytical of theoretical ideas, as well as enhancing the capacity of students and practitioners to generate professional knowledge – the distinction used by Elliott & Ebbutt (1985) between 'knowledge appliers' and 'knowledge generators'.

Reflection and reflective practice is currently of great interest to nurses, and the arrival of this book is an extremely timely event. In staying true to the tenets of the philosophical ideas that underpin reflection and reflective practice, the book is a useful mix of 'knowledge applied' and 'knowledge generated'. As is stated by the authors reflection is not the panacea for all ills, but it may help to address some of the criticisms that are levelled at nurse education and its 'product' – the trained professional nurse.

The so-called theory-practice gap has been a constant source of criticism for those practitioners and managers who are delivering the service, and from students who are experiencing it. The focus on learning from reflective processes has the potential to enhance and illuminate the realities of the context in which practice takes place, and to help the students and practitioners to describe and understand their own feelings and influence in the situation.

In relation to the development and delivery of health and social services, nursing has been seen to focus its attention at the level of individual client and patient, and to avoid or ignore the wider sociopolitical context of the health economy both at local organization level, and on the wider government or policy level. This has been seen to reflect a powerless nursing body which has little influence on the policy makers. There is potential through critical reflection and action, for students and practitioners to challenge the 'existing order' through an understanding of the factors which are influential beyond and outside their immediate situations (McTaggart 1993). These and many other issues are addressed in this book, which demonstrates very effectively that through a scholarly approach to educating nurses, the student's commitment to authentic practice is enhanced, resulting in a self-aware practitioner who can function with warmth, care, and critical enquiry.

References

Elliott, J. & Ebbutt, D. (1985) *Issues in teaching for understanding.* Longmans, for Schools Council, Harlow.

McTaggart, R. (1993) Dilemmas in cross cultural action research. In *Health Research in Practice*, (Eds. D. Colquhoun and A. Kellehear), Chapman and Hall, London.

Introduction

Today's nurses, more than at any other time, are faced with an increasing obligation to evaluate and improve their practice. The motivation to improve an individual's nursing practice may arise as an internal crusade, or it may emanate from external sources such as their peer group, their professional body or it could be politically driven. However, one thing remains clear – it is affecting, and no doubt should affect, each and every registered nurse, midwife and health visitor, regardless of where they practise, or how long they have practised. Yet nursing in our present climate often does not appear to foster professional self-evaluation. One of the many reasons for this could be the result of nursing in the 1990s which appears to be more akin to competing in a race rather than providing client centred, holistic health care. For many nurses, midwives and health visitors survival involves switching to autopilot just to complete the myriad tasks which are part of professional practice (Street, 1991). There are, however, real problems associated with switching to autopilot, the most important being that when a practitioner fails to consider his or her practice in a thoughtful and critical way, the individual needs of the client may not be met. This may lead to professionals who will increasingly alienate themselves from their clients and their colleagues in order to survive the trials of practice.

The concept of reflective practice is emerging as a means of addressing the alienation brought about by the 'high speed' manner in which nurses are expected to care for their clients. It is a concept that so far has not been rigorously tested or validated in nursing practice. Yet, despite this, reflection as a process for examining nurses' actions has been steadily gathering momentum throughout the United Kingdom. It is timely therefore for a textbook which devotes itself to exploring this concept, and the potential of reflection for developing nurses and their practice. This book has been written by nurses, primarily for nurses. However, in the development of this book it has become clear that many of the concepts explored, the issues faced and the tentative solutions offered, are applicable to many other professions which offer a service to clients who are vulnerable, or whose position in society is compromised. I therefore envisage that this book will be equally useful to other professionals.

Reflection in nursing is seen as a way to:

> 'Empower nurses to become fully cognizant of their own knowledge and actions, the personal and professional histories which have shaped them, the symbols and images inherent in the language they use, the myths and the metaphors which sustain them in practice, their nursing experiences, and the potentialities and constraints of their work setting.'
>
> Street (1991) page 1.

Whilst this movement to develop the use of reflection in nursing is on the whole commendable, many senior nurses and managers of nurse education have little idea as to the range of complex issues involved in adopting reflective practice, nor are they aware of the effects this process can have on nursing students and practitioners alike.

The experience so far in Oxfordshire would suggest that it is much easier for students and practitioners to grasp a conceptual understanding of reflection, whereas it is inherently more difficult for practitioners to make the essential link between their conceptual understanding, and their work with clients. This will be explored further in some of the following chapters. Our purpose then is to communicate the knowledge and expertise which has been developing in Oxfordshire as a result of an innovative and exciting practice-led curriculum for undergraduate and more recently post-registration nurse education which fundamentally values and supports the development of the emerging reflective practitioner. Furthermore, we aim to explore underlying issues and problems, to describe a selection of initiatives and to fulfil a need for novice reflective practitioners to find out more about the processes involved.

As a novice reflective practitioner you may be a student nurse on a traditional registered nurse or midwifery programme. Alternatively you may be a Project 2000 or undergraduate student experiencing nursing for the very first time. However, it is also highly likely that you could be a registered nurse, a midwife, a health visitor, a nurse educator or a nurse manager considering and analysing your professional practice for your own personal development or possibly as part of a continuing education programme. This book attempts to demonstrate the important link between the theory and practice of reflection by exploring the issues which underpin its use and by analysing numerous examples which will serve to illustrate the various issues and processes involved. It is not expected that nurses reading this book will have prior knowledge of either the concept of reflection or will necessarily have experience of using reflection in clinical practice. This means that a number of the chapters in the book will be useful as an introduction.

The book consists of chapters on various aspects of reflection from contributors who are, essentially nurses, and who have, over recent years, themselves struggled to introduce reflection into their nursing practice and education. When this book was written all the contributors were either engaged in nursing practice or education, either as undergraduate nurses, primary nurses, lecturer-practitioners or lecturers. The motivation to write this book came from a strongly held belief that what we as nurses have achieved so far with the concept of reflective practice, needs to be shared and explored with a wider nursing audience. This will enable the debate on the use of reflection to continue throughout the United Kingdom and beyond, and importantly, we hope that it will act as a catalyst for future research. Each of the contributors has adopted reflection as a way of improving their own professional practice. It must be stressed at the outset however that reflection is not, and will not be, a panacea for nursing. Nor will reflection provide the answers to the many difficult problems which face nursing as a developing profession. It is important, however, to consider and explore just what 'reflection' *can* offer the profession of nursing.

Following four years of using reflection with undergraduate nursing students and more recently with post-registration students, the experience so far suggests that reflection in the context of nurse education contains boundless opportunities for the profession to develop the competent, self-aware, analytical and confident clinical nurse practitioners of the future. Whereas in the past nurse educators have arguably not prepared students adequately for the rigours they face ahead as registered practitioners, reflection when integrated into the nursing curriculum and supported fully in practice may possibly prove to be the missing link to ensuring that what they learn in clinical practice is meaningful and valid to everyday practice. The power of reflection was brought home to me in one of my earliest experiences involving a nursing student who, while reflecting for her first ever day in clinical practice within a community hospital care of the elderly ward, documented in her learning contract the following experience:

'The importance of non-verbal communication was highlighted in the case of one very sick, terminally ill patient whom I came into contact with on my very first day. He was extremely weak and a chest infection made talking very difficult. He was also in great pain. When I was standing by his bedside, he grabbed hold of my hand really tightly. This may have been due to pain or simply the need to touch and make contact with another person. It would be sad if people in this condition were denied such contact in their last hours. This non-verbal communication may be the only type of contact between a dying patient and relatives – it can convey so much.

Later that same day I felt extremely inhibited when standing by the bedside of a severely brain damaged patient. As Margaret, my mentor, pointed out, we really don't know what is going on within that person; they may be aware of the situation around them. If this is so, talking to them is obviously important. I found it difficult to know what to say and was really conscious of others listening to me, thinking "why is she talking to him?".

Touch in this case was very important. Also when with this patient it was easy to ignore him and just chat to my other companions – this is something I must continually be aware of.'

What is so encouraging about this example is that it clearly demonstrates neophyte reflection, but importantly the reflection also demonstrates genuine compassionate caring *and* indicative learning. For this individual student the learning contract on which her personal learning is documented will remain a permanent reminder of her first ward experiences and as she progresses through her course of study it will record the continuing progress she makes, the feelings she experiences and some of the difficulties she encounters. As one can imagine, following the completion of a pre-registration programme of nurse education, this particular student will have amassed a prolific personal record of learning and achievement, and a powerful personal profile.

However we are not only concerned with nurse education and the preparation of the *future* nursing workforce but also today's nurses – the *current* nursing workforce.

To practise as a registered nurse, midwife or health visitor is comparable to practising in many other professional roles that involve dealing with vulnerable human beings. This professional work is frequently confusing and at times chaotic. Making sense of this chaos is not always easy. Even the most straightforward and simple procedure for such a professional can often become entangled with ambiguity and turmoil.

The following example illustrates this point:

It was 3 AM and Susan, a part-time registered nurse, discovered an elderly client's bed was wet with urine. The untrained nurse began to change and remake the bed whilst Susan began to prepare to remove the client's night-dress in order to clean her skin and replace the garment. Susan was about to remove the nightdress when the client yelled at her at the top of her voice to stop and hung on to her nightdress and cardigan as tightly as she could. Susan was alarmed and surprised at the reaction from the client. The client was cold and half asleep and wanted to get back into bed immediately. Susan began to explain to the client how important it was that her nightdress was removed when the client screamed: '*If you dare to touch my nightdress again I promise you I will scream this place down!*'

Susan felt terrible and to prevent the whole ward being woken up she proceeded to put the client back to bed with a slightly damp nightdress. For the remaining part of the night Susan worried constantly about how she could justify this action to the nurse in charge at handover the following morning.

For the nurses reading this example, it represents nothing unusual. There are numerous occasions in a nurse's professional life when things do not go as anticipated with a client, possibly more frequently than we sometimes would like to admit. When it happens, however, as the example so clearly illustrates, it is difficult to decide how to examine critically what exactly did happen. Furthermore, it makes it difficult to examine the situation in such a way that a positive learning outcome, in the form of professional growth, results. In the previous example it is shown that professional growth may be accomplished by reflecting on the standard of assessment, and on the implementation and evaluation of the decision making, which was a necessary element of the nursing action. This dynamic process will allow the practitioner ultimately to prepare for similar situations in the future as well as enable her carefully to unpick the various issues, conflicts and challenges which are entangled within the experience described. What is certain, in a profession such as nursing, is that no 'off the shelf' easy recipes exist, which will inform and direct nursing practice. What nurses are required to do, and must do therefore, is to begin to construct a personal database of knowledge which informs and enriches that individual's professional practice.

This book should help you to do just that. It will take you through the various stages of reflection and will enable you to make more sense of challenging clinical situations. The perspective of reality within the book will be immediately evident to the reader because the contributors are all writing from and about their personal experiences of using reflection in clinical, managerial, research or educational situations. There will be some amongst you who will feel that you reflect already and that you are already reviewing your practice. I hope this book challenges that assumption in a way that enables you to be more critical and allows thoughtful reflection to emerge. Reflection can be a difficult and frequently uncomfortable process. Saylor (1990) provides an illustrative example of a student teacher who is trying to master reflection.

'I've been thinking recently about how difficult it is to be reflective . . . I often feel like I don't have enough time to step back and evaluate how effective I am. By the time I finish one day, I usually feel like there is still next day's mountain to climb... Another thing about reflection – it's hard. It's hard because one must analyse what's transpired and to some degree, make a value judgement about it. And if the reflection is honest, it can mean that I may have to alter my style or completely chuck something that I have worked hard to develop. It seems to be much safer and secure not to reflect, because I don't have to change that which I don't see as wrong.'

Saylor (1990) p. 11.

There are a number of chapters within the book which also illustrate how difficult reflection can sometimes be in a nursing context. Some of the examples contained within the book are those of registered practitioners and students who have found it desperately hard to question their own practice in a critical way when it has been safer to avoid doing so. I believe Saylor's student teacher example has unmistakable parallels with nursing. Nurses today experience similar pressures working within a health service ethos which encourages both the performance of standard procedures and efficiency (Jarvis, 1992).

Thus the future implementation and success of reflection may to some extent rely on whether the organization allows reflection to occur. However, if reflective practice offers a possible solution to the current competency debate, then do nurses have a moral responsibility to begin to work towards becoming reflective practitioners? This argument is not as clear as it may seem. On the one hand, the first three points outlined in the revised UKCC Code of Professional Conduct (1992) leave us in no doubt about what we should do:

(1) Act in such a manner as to promote and safeguard the interests and well being of patients and clients;
(2) Ensure that no action or omission on your part, or within your sphere of responsibility, is detrimental to the interests, condition or safety of patients and clients;
(3) Maintain and improve your professional knowledge and competence.

UKCC Code of Professional Conduct (1992)

It could be suggested from the extract of the revised UKCC Code of Professional Conduct (1992), that it will be the responsibility of each practising nurse, midwife, and health visitor to introduce reflection into their professional practice if reflection is considered a necessary requisite for the evaluation and development of professional practice. On the other hand, do the conditions of practice allow for reflection to take place and is it therefore reasonable to expect nurses to take this concept on board? To enable the concept of reflection to develop, particularly within the National Health Service, it will be important that structures exist and 'professional space' is made available for the individual practitioner to reflect. Perhaps an example will illustrate this point.

The drive for efficiency and cost effectiveness within health services often leaves little time for an individual nurse or group of nurses to reflect on their clinical practice. The changes over recent years to the hospital midday shift overlap serves as a useful example. There has been a significant trend by managers of health care to reduce the handover time between the early and the late nursing shift. This has been primarily financially driven in an attempt to reduce nursing costs as it is suggested that this overlap represents a waste of nursing resources which could be more effectively deployed at other times of day (Stilwell & Hawley, 1993). Many wards and departments as a result of these cutbacks are left with a nursing handover time of no more than one hour. The effects of these handover cutbacks are only now becoming clear. In a major Welsh study into the management of nursing resources in acute hospitals a team of researchers looked closely at 14 wards with overlaps of different lengths, from one hour to three hours (Stilwell & Hawley, 1993). They concluded:

(1) The length of time when extra staff were on duty did not differ greatly between the wards with long overlaps and those with short overlap periods.
(2) On wards with long overlap periods, the effects of part-time staff, allocated half days and meal breaks resulted in *fewer* staff being present in the overlap period compared to the rest of the day. Thus the potential for making time available for 'extras' and personal activities was lost.
(3) On wards with short overlap periods the work with clients continued at a frenetic pace and opportunities for private study and teaching learners were lost.

The organization in which nurses work therefore appears to be a crucial factor if they are to take up the concept of reflective practice realistically. An organization which encourages reflection in its practitioners must, I believe, value the professional contribution that each and every practitioner makes. In addition the leaders within that organization must also desire that each and every practitioner has the opportunity to reach his or her potential. This demands a clear commitment to the development of practice. I believe that in Oxfordshire we have that leadership as well as an increasing commitment throughout the organization to develop professional nursing.

Education will also play a key part if the concept of reflection is to be adopted fully into the nursing profession. Everyday nursing practice establishes knowledge, understanding and ideas about being a nurse. Therefore practice must be central to nurse education rather than peripheral to it. Nursing education must ensure that students learn from their clinical experience; it is this clinical experience which always provides one of the greatest challenges for nurse educators. It will therefore require nurse teachers and mentors in the classroom and clinical settings, who themselves are able to reflect, to ensure the preparation of future competent reflective practitioners. Educators therefore need to become well versed in the use of reflection because if students are to be encouraged to engage in reflective practice their educators must do likewise in order that they may also re-examine their own beliefs and practices.

Reflection demands not only time, but a safe environment. A safe environment refers to one in which nurses, caring about each other, can think about and discuss their work. Nurses needs support and encouragement to share their perceptions and concerns about nursing care without fear of adverse judgement. The long term effects of using reflection remain unclear. We hope this book stimulates research into reflection/reflective practice, in particular to uncover the knowledge which is embedded in everyday nursing practice. Traditionally such knowledge has remained uncharted and unstudied because as Benner (1984) points out, the differences between practical and theoretical knowledge have often been misunderstood.

In Oxfordshire we are very committed to the concept of reflective practice, not only in undergraduates, but also in qualified staff. Firstly Oxford is pushing back the boundaries in the way it assesses students in practice. We have, since 1990, begun the process of grading the students on their ability to reflect on their clinical experiences. This is facilitated through the use of learning contracts. Secondly, there is an increasing trend to incorporate supervised reflection into clinical units as one way of developing therapeutic nursing in its practitioners, (see Chapter 8 by Christopher Johns).

The interest in reflection will, I believe, intensify as the impact of mandatory re-registration with evidence of professional development, occurs in the near future. There will be a need to scrutinize and evaluate clinical learning processes at all levels within the organization to ensure more effective approaches and outcomes. Thus the concept is not limited to pre-registration courses; we are now beginning to incorporate reflection in Oxford into a variety of our post-registration courses such as the Diploma in Higher Education for registered nurses. There is undoubtedly a great deal of work that needs to be undertaken to assess whether the concept of reflection will be crucial to the future development of nursing or whether it turns out to be a complete red herring. I believe evidence suggests that reflection has caught on in nursing, and that it is slowly gathering momentum.

Finally, this book is essentially one to dip into. It is not intended that you, the reader, begin at Chapter 1 and proceed through the various chapters in a mechanical way. Rather we expect that you will actively seek out particular areas of interest. For those who would prefer to begin at Chapter 1 and then proceed through the chapters, we have tried to place each chapter in what we believe is a logical sequence of development.

References

Benner, P. (1984) *From Novice to Expert: Excellence and Power in Clinical Nursing Practice.* Addison-Wesley Publishing Company, California.

Jarvis, P. (1992) Reflective practice and nursing. *Nurse Education Today,* **12**, 174–81.

Saylor, C.R. (1990) Reflection and professional education: art, science, and competency. *Nurse Educator,* **15**, No. 2, March/April.

Stilwell, J.A. & Hawley, C. (1993) The costs of nursing care. *Journal of Nursing Management.* **1**, No. 1, January.

Street, A. (1991) *From Image to Action – Reflection in Nursing Practice.* Deakin University, Geelong.

UKCC (1992) *Code of Professional Conduct for the Nurse, Midwife and Health Visitor,* 2nd edn, June. United Kingdom Central Council for Nursing, Midwifery and Health Visiting, London.

Chapter 1
Reflection with a Practice-Led Curriculum

Introduction

Within nursing there has recently been a growing interest in how professionals learn. Practitioners face challenging and unique situations within practice and need flexible ways of responding to and learning from these situations. Many courses have not prepared practitioners to meet such challenges (UKCC, 1986). The gaps between theory and practice and the rigid application of scientific approaches have not been conducive to preparing competent professional practitioners (Melia (1987), Champion (1992)).

The need for practice to be at the centre of professional learning is being acknowledged (Bines & Watson, 1992). Without this focus on practice it is unlikely that the skills required for competent practice will be developed. It is therefore essential that approaches which facilitate learning through practice are considered. While many courses have incorporated periods in practice in their curricula, this does not necessarily develop competence. It is not enough just to be practising; being there does not necessarily equal learning. The need for a tool which practitioners can use to facilitate learning through practice is crucial. One such tool which may enable effective learning from practice is reflection. The focus on practice and the incorporation of reflection as a learning tool demand new approaches to curriculum design and generate curricula which are practice-led. Innovative courses centred in practice have been developed (Champion, 1992) and demonstrate the potential of practice-led curricula.

The nature of professional education

Professional education is about preparing practitioners for, and supporting them in, their practice. Jarvis (1983) suggests that professional education should facilitate the development of a professional ideology, and provide students with opportunities to develop the knowledge and skills required for competent practice. Boud *et al.* (1985) expand upon these ideas, arguing that competency involves not only taking action in practice but learning from practice through reflection. Competence, standards of practice and the expectations of the public are considered by Watson (1992) as necessary concerns for those involved in professional education. At the heart of professional education therefore, is the aim of developing practitioners who are competent and who can respond to changing needs in the world of practice.

In many professional education courses the focus has been on enabling students to develop competencies. This focus is important because it places practice at the centre of the educational process, and by engaging professionals in an analysis of practice it may further understanding. Developing competence therefore is an important and integral component of professional education. Central to competence is the need to prepare practitioners who are capable of responding to and learning from unique situations in practice and who are able to develop further their professional expertise. This is supported by Schien (1972) who argues that at the centre of professional competence lies the capacity to 'learn how to learn'.

In discussing issues in professional education it has been claimed that some schools do not produce competent practitioners (Boud *et al.*, 1985). Two reasons are put forward. First, that professional schools may not be helping professionals develop the real skills required for competence. Not only are competencies often difficult to articulate and specify but practice is essentially individual in its nature. It must be questioned whether it is possible to specify general competencies which remain relevant to unique and indeterminate situations of practice. Second, in the changing world of practice, the skills required for competence may also change. The skills which represent competence today may be quite different from those required tomorrow.

While these issues are of significance for those involved in professional education in general, a particular concern in nursing education has been the perceived gap between the theory and practice of nursing. Studies by Bendall (1975), Melia (1987), Gott (1984) and Alexander (1983) have indicated that theory as taught in schools of nursing was not sufficiently related to practice. Gott (1984) concluded that nurse education programmes were failing to prepare student nurses for what was expected of them in clinical practice. Melia (1987) suggested that nurse education provided students with an idealized theoretical view of nursing which failed to prepare students for 'getting the work done'. These problems were compounded by the fact that many clinical environments were not conducive to learning (Fretwell (1982), Orton (1983), Ogier (1982), Reid (1985)). A serious question must therefore arise as to whether a two step approach of developing knowledge/theory within the classroom and then applying it to practice, in areas that may not be conducive to professional learning, can really develop the skills required to respond to unique practice situations. Growing dissatisfaction with the apparent inability of nurse education programmes to develop the skills required for practice has been mirrored by a similar discontent within other professional groups. This has given rise to a debate about the nature of professional education.

Schön (1983), in exploring the nature of professional practice, suggests that professionals are faced with situations of uncertainty, instability and complexity which are unique and insoluble by the strict application of technical rational approaches.

Bines (1992) identifies the elements of technical rationality as the development of research based empirical knowledge, and the application of this knowledge in a supervised practice placement. Schön (1983) suggests that a focus on technical rationality fails to reflect the fundamental nature of professional knowledge and action, and the ways in which professionals develop their practice. Bines (1992) argues that most professional activity is not based on learning knowledge and applying it in practice but on an integrated knowledge-in-action approach, much of which is spontaneous and tacit. Therefore empirical knowledge alone may not be sufficient for professional practice which, because it involves interaction with people, is inherently unique, individual and complex.

Some authors (e.g. Carper (1978), Benner & Tanner (1987)) have identified other types of knowledge used in nursing practice. Carper (1978) showed that nurses use aesthetic, moral and personal knowledge in addition to empirical knowledge. Benner & Tanner (1987) in particular emphasize the importance of intuitive knowledge. It is important therefore that nursing education should offer opportunities for learning in all these spheres of knowledge. Clearly, if professional education programmes focus exclusively on the development of technical rational knowledge they may not be developing in practitioners the ability to solve practice problems.

To enable practitioners to develop the skills required for practice, Schön (1991) advocates a model of professional learning where professionals learn by reflecting within a practicum. It is important therefore to examine the nature of reflection and the features of a practicum.

Nature of reflection

Boyd & Fales (1983) offer a useful definition of reflection, suggesting that it is:

'The process of internally examining and exploring an issue of concern, triggered by an experience, which creates and clarifies meaning in terms of self, and which results in a changed conceptual perspective'

Reflection is initiated by an awareness of uncomfortable feelings and thoughts which arise from a realization that the knowledge one was applying in a situation was not itself sufficient to explain what was happening in that unique situation. The focus of learning is upon critical analysis of these unique practice situations. It is important that this analysis involves an examination of both feelings and knowledge so that the knowledge required for professional practice is illuminated. This may include aesthetic, personal, moral as well as empirical knowledge. In addition, because reflection involves exploration of a unique situation, new knowledge may be generated. Reflection therefore has the potential to address the problems of practice in a way that the application of technical rational approaches alone do not.

Schön (1991) distinguishes between two types of reflection: reflection-in-action and reflection-on-action. Reflection-in-action occurs while practising, and influences the decisions made and the care given, whereas reflection-on-action occurs after the event and contributes to the development of practice skills. Practitioners learn from both types of reflection and these need to be facilitated within a practice-led curriculum. Learning by reflection can be facilitated most effectively within a practicum.

Features of a practicum

The features of a practicum have been discussed by Schön (1983, 1987) and Bines (1922). A practicum is a structured environment where students, supported by experienced practitioners, are encouraged to reflect upon simulated or actual practice situations. The practicum is the key and integrating element of professional education. The practicum should offer conditions of safety to the learner which enable him or her to explored dilemmas and to become aware of the defences which may inhibit their growth or that of others.

Argyris & Schön (1974) argue that people work with two types of theories of action: espoused theories, which are used to explain or justify behaviour, and theories-in-use, which govern actual behaviours. Many people tend to keep their espoused theories and theories-in-use compartmentalized as they may not be congruent. Establishing a reflective practicum can create the conditions for exposing behaviours, allowing practitioners to become aware of their theories-in-use. Zeichner

(1990) suggests that organization and structure of the practicum are central to its success as a place of learning.

Designing a curriculum for professional education

From the arguments above it is evident that a focus on practice is the essential prerequisite of a professional course. Practice-led curricula therefore need to be generated. Bines (1992) argues that there are two key issues in course design, the aims of the course and how those aims are realized. When using a model of professional education, course aims can only be realized if the curriculum is practice-led.

Bines (1992) identifies three models of professional education: the pre-technocratic, the technocratic and the post-technocratic. The pre-technocratic model largely comprises the acquisition of skills through on-the-job training with theoretical instruction during block or day release. This is largely an apprenticeship model of training, and has been the dominant model of nurse education prior to Project 2000 programmes.

In contrast, the technocratic model is characterized by three elements. First the development and transmission of systematic knowledge, based upon contributing academic disciplines. Second, the interpretation and application of that knowledge to practice. Third, supervised practice in selected placements. This model is the one largely adopted by nurse education programmes integrated into higher education.

Traditionally nursing has depended upon the bio-medical model which is firmly rooted in the scientific method and the scientific philosophies (Clarke, 1986). Therefore the technocratic model was appealing to nurses keen to gain academic credibility for nursing and to establish a body of research knowledge related to nursing. However, there are problems with this model. Not only does it fail to reflect the true nature of professional education, but it can lead to fragmentation of learning and dysfunction between theory and practice (Bines, 1992). Therefore the use of a technocratic model for curriculum development may in itself contribute to the gaps between theory and practice.

A more appropriate model for professional education may be the post-technocratic model. In this model, practice is the key place where competence is developed. Systematic reflection is used as a learning tool and skilled practitioners act as facilitators. In addition, course elements outside practice situations will also be focused on issues of professional practice.

If curricula are developed using this model, teaching and learning should be concerned with the development of professional knowledge, competence, and reflection. Practice becomes central and the gap between theory and practice minimalized. Support for a practice-led model has also come from French & Cross (1992). They argue for an interpersonal-epistemological curriculum model for nurse education. This shares some of the features of the post-technocratic approach and focuses on forms of knowledge and interpersonal relationships. They share an emphasis on the need to develop both the practicum and reflective skills.

Making a practice-led curriculum work

In order for a practice-led curriculum to be effective, attention needs to be given to developing the practicum, to the teaching methods used and to the assessment strategies.

Developing the practicum

A practicum is by its nature an environment that is conducive to learning. It has been suggested that it should be safe, organized and structured in order to facilitate learning fully.

One approach to developing a practicum is through the employment of lecturer-practitioners. Lecturer-practitioners are senior practitioners with expertise in practice, management, education and research (Fitzgerald (1989), Vaughan (1990)). They can provide leadership in facilitating practice-based learning by helping students and professional practitioners develop reflective abilities. This is because they have the authority, responsibility and accountability for both standards of practice within their work area, and for contributing to the curricula of practice-based educational courses (Champion, 1992). Whilst their roles require further evaluation and clarification, the experiences of some lecturer-practitioners suggest that their value lies in the unified perspective they can bring to practice and education and in enabling professional education to be firmly rooted in practice (Lathlean (1992), Champion (1992)).

A further consideration in developing the practicum is the role of mentors. It is suggested that learning through experience and developing reflective abilities may be enhanced through individual supervision of learners by competent nurses acting as mentors (Burnard, 1989). Within nursing education, a formal pattern of mentoring is emerging whereby learners are assigned to experienced practitioners for the purpose of facilitating learning through practice (ENB (1989), Morris *et al.*, (1992)).

Mentors may be able to facilitate learning by articulating the knowledge behind their actions, and by promoting the use of reflection as a learning tool to study practice situations on a regular basis. The time taken to do this and the need for careful selection of mentors cannot be under-estimated. However, mentors are key people in supporting students and facilitating learning within the practicum (Atkins, 1992).

Structuring the practicum so that it is conducive to learning can, however, be resource intensive. Managers therefore need to see professional education as important and have a commitment to its development. The education of practitioners must be resourced accordingly.

Teaching and learning

If in a practice-led curriculum the focus is upon competence and the development of reflection then approaches to learning must be congruent with this. Student centred, facilitative styles of teaching may be most appropriate to enable the development of the skills required for competence and to use reflection as a learning tool (Champion, 1992). In particular the skills of self-awareness, description, critical analysis, synthesis and evaluation have been identified as necessary to engage in reflection (Atkins & Murphy, 1993).

Exploring feelings can be difficult and may leave the student feeling vulnerable. The practicum must provide conditions of safety, warmth and trust to enable students to undertake a full exploration of feelings. To utilize the potential of reflection as a learning tool, the course team must ensure that opportunities to develop these skills exist throughout the course.

In addition if learners are to develop the skills of lifelong learning, self-directed techniques and increasing student involvement in deciding and controlling the learning process appears appropriate (French & Cross, 1992).

Assessment

Appropriate thought must be given to assessing the development of competence within the practicum. If learning is centred in practice then it is important that students see this learning as significant and as contributing to their overall programme.

It may also be that students will be more motivated to learn in practice if that learning contributes significantly to their overall marks. Assessing and grading practice which focuses upon competence is not easy (Murphy & Reading (1992), Burns (1991)). Grading criteria need to be developed which are clear and unambiguous. Evidence of competence needs to be gathered in a way that allows moderation of, and debate about, the grades awarded. One potential way of gathering evidence of competence is through students' written accounts of practice situations, utilizing a reflective model.

Conclusions

The aim of professional education is clearly the development of practitioners who are competent and who can respond to changing needs in the world of practice. Practitioners require more than empirical knowledge for competence, and reflection has been demonstrated as a key tool for learning in practice situations. In order to make a practice-led curriculum work, the practicum must be safe, organized and structured, and this cannot be left to chance.

Lecturer-practitioners and mentors are essential to the effectiveness of the practicum, and the most appropriate teaching strategies are facilitative. It is clear therefore that effective professional education is resource intensive. Mentors and lecturer-practitioners require preparation for their roles, and time to fulfil these responsibilities. At a time when National Health Service resources are under strain and intense scrutiny, the need for this additional expense may appear difficult to justify. There may be those who argue that the time given to student learning is time taken away from client care. However, the long term benefits of developing reflective abilities and real competence in practitioners are worthy of serious consideration, and may ultimately be cost effective. Practitioners who have learned how to learn and who can respond to the unique challenges of practice may be more effective in meeting clients' needs.

References

Alexander, M.F. (1983) *Learning to Nurse: Integrating Theory and Practice*, Churchill Livingstone, Edinburgh.

Argyris, C. & Schön, D. (1974) *Theory in Practice: Increasing Professional Effectiveness*, Addison-Wesley, Massachusetts.

Atkins, S. (1992) *Registered nurses' experiences of mentoring undergraduate student nurses: a qualitative analysis.* MSc thesis, University of Manchester.

Atkins, S. & Murphy, K. (1993) Reflection: a review of the literature, *Journal of Advanced Nursing*, November 1992.

Bendall, E. (1975) *So, You Passed Nurse*, Royal College of Nursing, London.

Benner, P. & Tanner, C. (1987) Clinical judgement: how expert nurses use intuition, *American Journal of Nursing*, **87**(1), 23–31.

Bines, H. (1992) Issues in course design. In: *Developing Professional Education* (eds H. Bines & D. Watson), Society for Research into Higher Education and Open University Press, Buckingham.

Bines, H. & Watson, D. (1992) *Developing Professional Education*, Society for Research into Higher Education and Open University Press, Buckingham.

Boud, D., Keogh, R. & Walker, D. (1985) *Reflection: Turning Experience into Learning*, Kogan Page, London.

Boyd, E.M. & Fales, A.W. (1983) Reflecting learning: key to learning from experience, *Journal of Humanistic Psychology*, **23**(2), 99–117.

Burnard, P. (1989) *Counselling Skills for Health Professionals*. Chapman & Hall, London.

Burns, S. (1991) Grading Practice, *Nursing Times*, **88**(1), pp. 40–42.

Carper, B. (1978) Fundamental patterns of knowing in nursing, *Advances in Nursing Science*, **1**, 13–23.

Champion, R. (1992) The philosophy of an honours degree programme in nursing and midwifery. In: *Developing Professional Education* (eds H. Bines & D. Watson). Society for Research into Higher Education and Open University Press, Buckingham.

Clarke, M. (1986) Action and reflection: practice and theory in nursing. *Journal of Advanced Nursing*, **11**(1), 3–11.

ENB (1989) Preparation of Teachers, Practitioner Teachers, Mentors and Supervisors in the Context of Project 2000, English National Board, London.

Fitzgerald, M. (1989) *Lecturer-practitioner: action researcher*, MA thesis, University of Wales, School of Nursing.

French, P. & Cross, D. (1992) An interpersonal epistemological curriculum model for nurse education, *Journal of Advanced Nursing*, **17**, 83–9.

Fretwell, J. (1982) *Ward Learning and Teaching: Sister and the Learning Environment*, Royal College of Nursing, London.

Gott, M. (1984) *Learning Nursing*, Royal College of Nursing, London.

Jarvis, P. (1983) *Professional Education*, Croom Helm, London.

Lathlean, J. (1992) The contribution of lecturer-practitioners to theory and practice in nursing, *Journal of Clinical Nursing*, **1**, 237–42.

Melia, K. (1987) *Learning and Working – The Occupational Socialisation of Nurses*, Tavistock, London.

Morris, N., John, G. & Keen, T. (1992) Mentors learning the ropes, *Nursing Times*, **84** (46), 24–7.

Murphy, K. & Reading, P. (1992) Assessing professional competence. In: *Developing Professional Education*, (eds H. Bines & D. Watson), SRHE and Open University Press, Buckingham.

Ogier, M. (1982) *An Ideal Sister? A Study of Leadership Style and Verbal*

Interactions of Ward Sisters with Nurse Learners in General Hospitals, Royal College of Nursing, London.

Orton, H. (1983) *Ward Learning Climate*, Royal College of Nursing, London.

Reid, N. (1985) *Wards in Chancery? Nurse Training in the Clinical Area*, Royal College of Nursing, London.

Schien, E.H. (1972) Occupational Socialisation in the Professions: the case of role innovation. *Journal of Psychol. Research*, **8**, 521–30.

Schön, D.A. (1983) *The Reflective Practitioner*, Temple Smith, London.

Schön, D.A. (1987) *Educating the Reflective Practitioner*, Jossey Bass, London.

Schön, D.A. (1991) *The Reflective Practitioner*, 2nd edition, Temple Smith, London.

UKCC (United Kingdom Central Council for Nurses, Midwives and Health Visitors) (1986) *Project 2000: A New Preparation for Practice*, London.

Vaughan, B. (1990) Knowing that and knowing how: the role of the lecturer practitioner. In: *Models of Nursing 2*, (eds B. Kershaw & J. Salvage), Scutari Press, London.

Watson, D. (1992) The changing shape of professional education. In: *Developing Professional Education*, (eds H. Bines & D. Watson), SRHE and Open University Press, Buckingham.

Zeichner (1990) Changing directions in the practicum; looking ahead to the 1990s. *Journal of Education for Teaching*, **16**(2), 105–32.

Chapter 2
Assessing Reflective Learning

Introduction

This chapter seeks to explore the issues related to assessing learning from reflective processes. The argument is presented for assessing the process *and* outcome of learning from reflection, supporting the idea of integrating theory and practice in nursing within one assessment rather than separating the two and thus perpetuating the 'theory practice' gap. This is followed by description of one integrated assessment strategy currently used in an undergraduate nursing programme. The potential for such a strategy across post-registration education and the possibilities within the forthcoming mandatory registration are described. In conclusion key issues and implications for the future are discussed.

Why assess learning from reflective processes?

Darbyshire *et al.* (1990) suggested that we've not much to be proud of in the area of assessing the clinical practice of nurses. Alexander (1983), amongst others, finds this unacceptable and argues that clinical practice *and* theory should be given equal priority in any assessment. Why is it that we have had separate assessment of theory and practice? Have we been prevented by educational sophistication from seeing that we have been outcomes focused? Was it convenient to address outcomes assessment or was it the effect of the theory practice gap? The gap between theory and practice has been well documented over the years (Lathlean, 1992) and it is not viewed positively. Although some authors have made some tentative suggestions on how to eradicate it, little seems to have had an effect.

There are, however, two significant issues which will change this situation. Firstly, developments in clinical practice which support and enhance the nurse in giving patient centred care. Binnie & Titchen (1993) have highlighted the individualistic and humane approach developing in nursing. The increased value attached to the relationship between nurse and patient shows sensitivity and recognition of individual needs. This transition is supported by Bevis's (1978) analysis of the fundamental ideologies in nursing (see Fig. 2.1). As she traces the emerging ideologies over the last 200 years one can see clearly the recognition of the individual gaining credence in nursing at the end of the twentieth century. This recognition of the individual demands of the nurse skills in problem framing, decision making and communication.

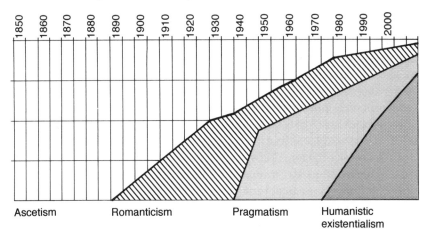

Fig. 2.1   Chronology of four philosophical systems which affect nursing (Bevis (1978)).

The second issue impacting on the theory practice gap is Project 2000 (UKCC, 1986) and the general revolution in nurse education that has taken place since 1988. New nursing curricula have been implemented nationwide. One common feature of these curricula is the description of the desirable features the exiting student should have. These written competencies and learning outcomes further define what this means in reality. The phrase *knowledgeable doer* is seen in a number of course philosophies. If the desirable outcome is a knowledgeable doer then assessment should be devised to determine this. Thus, assessment must be theory and practice combined.

What lessons, if any, can we learn from our past efforts at assessing learning in practice? The endless comments that it was (and perhaps is) horrendously difficult to do, and fraught with known and unknown pitfalls, seems to have influenced nurse educators in pursuing academically credible strategies for theoretical assessment at the expense of clinical assessment. Add to this the relatively few nurse educators who still have credible clinical skills themselves, and one can see some reasons for our dependence on outcome assessment rather than assessing the process as well. The impact of educators in practice, in the form of lecturer-practitioners is one way forward (Dearmun, 1993). The structure of lecturer-practitioners working in practice, alongside students and their mentors potentially allows assessment of both the *process* of students' learning as well as the product.

Reflective learning, as described in Chapter 1 allows for the contextual issues in practice to be acknowledged in learning experiences, therefore assessment of reflective learning should do as well. It is our challenge to develop assessment strategies supportive of this reflective learning.

If we accept the changing face of nursing practice and education and agree we need to expand our range of assessment tools then we can tackle the complexities of assessing clinical ability in a holistic way rather than as isolated competencies. Expecting students to pull competencies together and in the process somehow magically achieve knowledgeable doing is unacceptable. In using reflection in practice we have at last acknowledged the complex murky reality of clinical practice. The work of Schön (1983) and Boud *et al.* (1985) among others, has clearly been influential in enabling nursing to look confidently at its practice. It has been an almost inevitable consequence of the impact of humanistic ideology emerging in clinical practice (Bevis, 1978). This leads on to gradual recognition that we have perhaps overly depended on the outcome of learning measurement, as in competencies, rather than taken account of the process of learning. An exclusive focus on outcome measure is no longer acceptable. It does not adequately demonstrate the process by which the knowledgeable doer arrives at his/her actions/solutions. The knowledgeable doer has to be assessed in both process and outcome measures.

Requirements from both statutory and professional bodies have determined that some monitoring and achievement of standards in selection, preparation and registration of nurses is maintained. The current Nurses' and Midwives' Rules (UKCC, 1983) are statutory requirements for nurses seeking to register. In the form of competencies the Rules seek to make explicit the minimum standard of behaviour a registered nurse will exhibit. The consequence of such an outcome focused approach is that the essence of the whole which is greater than the sum of the parts is lost. It is not simply the total of skills achieved separately that will determine the knowledgeable doer but rather the effective use of clusters of competencies that the student uses in clinical situations. The ability to be flexible and adaptable without losing sight of purpose, to be able to work *with* human individuality rather than *against* it is what we are striving to develop in the nurse for the year 2000 and beyond.

What can be or should be assessed from reflective learning?

As determined in the previous section it is both the process and outcome of learning from reflection that are to be assessed. First outcome; this is described in the form of competencies. The definitive list of competencies was determined by a group of nurse practitioners and educators at Oxford Brookes University. The group used the work of Carper (1978), Benner (1984) and the Nurses and Midwives Rules (1983) as a framework and determined competencies at four levels, to correspond roughly with the four years of the degree programme. For example:

Level 1   Recognizes own beliefs and values and the effect of these on self and own behaviour

Level 2   Explores some of the implications of own beliefs and values as a student of nursing and midwifery

Level 3   Analyses the nature of moral/ethical issues and contributes to discussion in clinical practice

Level 4   Contributes to ethical decision making about client care

With this framework of competencies the outcome behaviours were identified. In assessment terms pass/fail could now be determined. However, as indicated earlier, if the process of learning could somehow be made explicit, then the confidence of determining quality of practice, incorporating the theory underpinning the practice could be assessed.

The second strand was how to get the process presented for assessment. In both nursing and general education the use of learning contracts is widely accepted and increasingly used as a mechanism for students both to determine their own learning objectives and then to provide evidence to support the achievement or otherwise of learning (Bines & Watson (1992), Jarvis (1992)). A relatively simple design was devised so as to maximize student individuality. We agreed on a contract that had four columns only: learning objectives, resources, and strategies, evidence and reflection, and validation. The validation column is important to include so that any experience offered for assessment is validated as an accurate description of what went on; validated by the student's mentor (see Chapter 3: The Mentor's Experience) or the lecturer-practitioner, both of whom work in clinical practice with the student and are therefore well placed to carry out this function. The contract design allows students to show their achievement of clinical competence by inviting reflection and analysis of the clinical experience which they feel best demonstrates this achievement.

Students are free to determine their learning objectives and the resources and strategies they will employ in trying to achieve their objectives. Students are assisted in this by using the written aims and focus of the area of learning to be addressed. In the undergraduate programme these are modules of 120–240 hours of work focusing on specific subject areas, for example, on Acute and Crisis Care or The Management of Adult Nursing. Students also use their mentor and their lecturer-practitioner in exploring learning objectives and resources and strategies. These people are best able to identify likely learning opportunities within the clinical area. Students then reflect on their learning and often record many of the details in personal journals (this is discussed further in Chapter 7 on students' experiences and Chapter 8 on supervision). Discussions with their mentor about the experience helps widen and deepen their understanding and provokes new areas to explore both in their reading and practice. A judiciously edited experience is then presented in the evidence and reflection column. This should demonstrate the competency achievement and the quality or nature of reflection the student has engaged in. Thus the process the student has been through in determining his or her action is evidenced and presented for assessment. The potential for grading this work therefore comes from the quality of reflection and not only the achievement of competence.

A pass is secured by demonstrating competence, the grade comes from the quality or level of reflection. It is important to reiterate that grading is determined by the quality of the reflection not the competence.

The work of Goodman (1984) and Mezirow (1981) amongst others, was helpful in determining possible grading criteria. Both of these writers in some way discriminate reflection into levels, Goodman into three broad levels, Mezirow into seven (see Chapter 5 for further discussion). These levels are helpful in determining the quality – or indeed existence – of higher order academic skills such as analysis or critical thinking which need to be determined in assessing degree level work.

Goodman (1984) describes three levels of reflection: reflection concerned with the techniques and practices needed to reach determined objectives; reflection on the relationship between practice and principles; and reflection building on this by developing an awareness of the ethical and political influences. Grade C or pass is determined by achievement of critical competencies for the relevant module of learning. Grades B, B+ and A are determined by the quality of reflection using Goodman's levels as the discriminating factors. Profiles of each of these grades have been explicitly written out and so are available to all students and stand for all learning contract grades, across modules, fields and years.

The first level is where reflection is mainly descriptive. Also the objectives have been determined largely by others and are not questioned by the student, where reflection is written in 'fly on the wall' style rather than as an active participant. There is limited, if any, acknowledgement of personal feelings and thoughts. For example:

'I asked her if she would like a wash – and she lit up at this proposition. I walked her down the corridor – as she said that she didn't feel stable enough to walk unaided. She happily went to the loo alone – whilst I ran some water for her in the bathroom sink and set her toiletries around the sink to make a bit of a fuss to cheer her up. She managed to wash unaided but needed help putting on a new clean nightdress. I made a fuss of her nice Avon toiletries and commented on how lovely she smelt to make her feel special and encourage her to be hygienic – to reinforce positive health behaviour.'

In this excerpt there is little evidence of clear thought – on the one hand the patient indicates she feels unsteady but the student makes no response other than to comment that she goes to the loo unaided.

Some evidence presented in contracts does indicate competence in a particular situation. However it does raise the issue of how transferable to another situation is this competence. Goodman's (1984) second level of reflection builds on this and calls for the reflection to show awareness of the implications of both personal and professional values and beliefs in relation to actions and to make explicit the rationales which govern actions. This clearly moves us into the area of the practitioner transferring competence across situations by clearly indicating the understanding behind the action taken.

The third level of reflection described by Goodman includes, in addition to the above, the acknowledgement of wider influences in the form of ethical and political concerns. Such reflection allows for understanding of how broader social forces, such as health policy, influence an individual in the course of their work.

The following excerpt from a third year adult nursing student's contract may help illustrate the level. The student is on placement in a hospice and had previously described her experiences feeding a patient (Jean) explaining how it was more than physically feeding but involved working at Jean's pace, using silence and being with her. She goes on to discuss:

'Bradley & Edinburg (1990) discuss the idea of nursing task visibility, classing nursing actions as either high visibility (task orientation) or low visibility (patient oriented) or both. A high visibility task is one which is more easily seen by other people e.g. setting up an IVI [Intravenous infusion]. It requires manual skill (physically doing something!) and is usually related to physio- logical functioning. A low visibility task cannot be seen easily by others, it requires cognitive/affective skill and is usually related to psychological needs of the patient. In other ward placements I have observed a very great emphasis on physical care (high visibility tasks) often resulting in the neglect of psychological care, ... to the casual observer (and maybe even professional observers) it might at times appear that the nurses on the ward did not have much work to do, that it was not a busy shift, e.g. because the nurse was able to sit out in the garden with a patient. This is the problem with low visibility nursing tasks (which much of palliative nursing care may be classed as – the work involves an emotional labour rather than a physical labour. What goes on is difficult to describe (almost invisible) and so is often devalued (Lawler, 1991). Also because there is the belief that "nursing skills are the refinement of the natural talents of women this too leads to the devaluing of nursing care" (Lawler). In the latter, care is not just the emotional labour but also the physical labour of body care. I am still learning to fully appreciate the importance and value of the work we do as nurses and nursing students – particularly the emotional work – on its own and as an important aspect of physical work. After a shift during which I cared for Jean I met up with a friend who asked "Well what did you do on the ward today?" I thought about this and replied "I fed a patient" – how simplistic. Although my friend was a fellow nursing student I felt unable (at the time) to express what I had put into this interaction and how I felt it was of benefit to the patient. Yet if we do not value what we do why should anyone else?

In assessing the level of reflection the incident (necessarily truncated for inclusion here) has been explored widely using associated reading to illuminate her actions. However the ruminations are clearly brought to personal level at the end of the excerpt.

How is assessment of learning from reflection carried out?

The starting point for us was the course philosophy statement which is included in the submission document for the ENB (Oxford Polytechnic (1986) p. 64).

'the analysis ... of the student's own work and the acceptance of new solutions arrived at by examining practice problems in a new light is seen as fundamental to the development of the emergent reflective professional.' (p. 67).

With such a clear statement we were then in a position to see what assessment tools could reasonably be used in the programme and where perhaps we needed to develop our own.

To some extent the procedure of assessment has been alluded to in the earlier part of this chapter but it is perhaps helpful to describe the procedure as a whole at this point. It is important to give enough background information about the course in general so that you are in a position to critically review this procedure with your own experiences/constraints etc.

The course is a four year programme preparing students for professional registration in either adult, paediatric, mental health, learning disabilities or midwifery with a BA (Hons) degree. The course is modular, with 29 modules combining with average marks leading to degree classification. Half the modules are clinically based and in support of the course philosophy are graded so as to allow clinical ability to be included in determining the degree classification as with theoretically based degrees. If the practice modules were not assessed in this way the final degree classification would be based on theoretical work and would not necessarily reflect the student's ability in practice.

All practice modules include part or total assessment using a learning contract as described previously. Each module is required to have a handbook outlining all pertinent information related to the content. Students determine their learning objectives using the module focus described within the module handbook. This is further amplified in discussion with the mentor and/or lecturer-practitioner from the clinical placement. As the module progresses, the student gains experience to help achieve competence and the chosen learning objective. Evidence is written in the contract. As the term progresses it is important that feedback is given by the lecturer-practitioner and mentor on the reflection demonstrated.

Reflective conversations between the student and mentor help widen the perspectives on any situation and encourage the student to look further into issues, as further relevant reading or associated issues which impinge on the understanding of the situation can be identified. Evidence of a dialogue between student and mentor via the validation column is clearly indicative of the process of learning. It is also a direct challenge to students who persist in seeing the superficial details of practice without clearly demonstrating the deeper understanding required of the knowledgeable doer.

At the end of the module the student is required to present the completed contract with validation from the mentor to the lecturer-practitioner for the grading viva. At this meeting student, mentor and lecturer-practitioner discuss aspects of the contract. While being put on the spot is daunting for all concerned, it has helped students and mentors to really appreciate the reflective process. Mentors may advocate on behalf of students and students may clarify entries and understandings when questioned. Lecturer-practitioners need to be sure of their ground, to have taken time to review the contract and be able to pose questions to the student to help illuminate the process, particularly with those students who encounter difficulties in getting to grips with it. Students are asked to self grade the contract along with suggested grades from the mentor and lecturer-practitioner. Discussions follow to find an agreeable mark which is then entered subject to the moderation process. Where agreement cannot be reached then the contract is put forward for further grading at moderation. Any changes to the grade made at moderation are clearly explained in writing on the grading comments sheet.

Moderation of the learning contract is vitally important in the process of assessment. Other assessors should review the work in order to counter the impact of subjective or personal bias entering into the process. The moderation process has been, and is, an intensively resourced part of the assessment process. This may be in part due to the learning required by the educators in getting to grips with a new process. However it is also important to assure students that they have not been advantaged or disadvantaged by their personal relationships with mentor and/or lecturer-practitioner. Moderation also allows for vindication of professional judgment in assessment. It is sound to use professional judgment (Brykczynki (1989), Hepworth (1989)), but others find it hard to trust it entirely (Newell, 1992), preferring objective evidence to be presented as well. The reality is that there are rarely significant differences in grading the same work. They do occasionally occur and this seriously challenges lecturer-practitioners to explore their own values and judgments in relation to clinical work, particularly their understanding of the grading criteria and their maturity in assessing work of people they know well at degree level.

Post-registration education assessment possibilities

The format described in the previous section relates to an undergraduate programme. In this section the issues of how an assessment strategy might be developed for registered nurses are explored.

The key difference to acknowledge is that post-registered students already know quite a lot about their nursing but have also recognized a need or wish to take their learning further. Also, many nurses feel that they already reflect on their practice though perhaps not as formally as reflective learning suggests, i.e. writing journals or reflective diaries – perhaps more with a stiff gin and tonic after work with a couple of friends discussing the rigours of the previous shift. The use of a learning contract within post-registration courses is appropriate as it allows each student to identify his or her own learning objectives. Students need guidance in identifying appropriate areas to learn about in relation to the focus of the course subject being studied. For example, post-registration diplomas in palliative, community and critical care identify competency outcomes of learning. While this is perhaps straightforward for students, as it mirrors approaches they have experienced in the past, the effort required in exploring the higher levels of reflection is more challenging. Some teaching teams have allowed for an introductory period with formative feedback initially as students develop an impression of what reflective, writing and analytical skills might be in relation to assessment by learning contract. In essence the process transfers well with recognition of the differing entry skills post-registered students have.

Forthcoming mandatory re-registration possibilities

Described so far has been the formal assessment of learning from reflection within pre- and post-registration courses. Learning from reflection for all nurses as Chapter 8, which gives the practitioner's perspective, clearly demonstrates, has tremendous potential. This is particularly pertinent as the profession moves towards mandatory re-registration with evidence of learning (UKCC, 1990). Shortly, all nurses seeking to re-register will be required to submit evidence of continued learning. The development of personal profiles or portfolios is being widely debated as a mechanism to provide this evidence.

Where and how might reflective learning evidence be included? It would seem quite reasonable that evidence in the form of a learning contract, for example, be included in a portfolio. The issues of validation might need further work, with some guidelines from the UKCC as to who might validate being helpful. However, the possibilities of peer or client validation should not be excluded. Overdependence on currently acceptable validators in the form of qualified teachers etc or specially trained assessors may make the process unwieldy and even denigrate the value of the work by missing out the key receivers of individuals' work, namely clients and colleagues.

Implication in practice

A number of issues arise from assessing learning from reflection. This is perhaps best reviewed by looking at the key personnel involved:

Students

Students have commented on their experiences with assessment of reflective learning in the following ways. Firstly, the uncertainty of using an unfamiliar learning approach. The lack of clear guidelines about how to complete work, to get even an idea of how the work is to be put together generated a significant amount of frustration, even anger for some. Students have been uncertain of their work, seeking clear guidelines that staff were either unwilling or unable to give. Unwilling, in that direct guidelines or examples for students to look at might result in very similar work being presented, which did not necessarily reflect how students might determine their own approach. Unable to give advice because they had no concrete experience of this process to share with students.

A second feature is the inconsistency students perceive in teaching staff both in relation to what was expected within contracts and in grading. Inconsistencies in advice resulted from teaching staff being wary of giving too much advice lest it be directive and inhibit students' interpretations or giving advice which reflected the more traditional approaches they were familiar with and so was not now appropriate. Students on the receiving end of this advice then became confused when such approaches were not rewarded in their grades. However the challenge has made us look harder at whether it is acceptable to rely on what is essentially professional judgment in the provision of clinical care. The grading criteria and competencies are reviewed regularly and documentation in the form of guidelines has been developed for students, mentors and lecturer-practitioners. As Long (1976) and Hepworth (1989) indicate, in the right circumstances professional judgment is reliable. Those circumstances include recognition of the context in which the activity was carried out. In using the learning contract students are able to describe the context and its impact on the situation. Also the validator, i.e. mentor, is in practice alongside the student, so is also aware of the relevant contextual issues impinging on the situation and the student's performance. Thus the validation of student competency and grading of reflection is reasonable. Informing the students of the reasoning behind the processes adopted is important. There may still however be inconsistencies of marking and these must be taken seriously. The extensive moderation procedures adopted help identify problems. Experience of marking across and within fields (i.e. are third year midwives and mental health students assessed to the same level) suggests significant consistency in marking. However, inexperienced teachers have been shown to be high markers so it is important that a clear introduction to the marking process and criteria is available for all staff new to the process.

Mentors

A key person in the assessment process is the student's mentor. Indeed the validity of the whole process is called into question if no mentor is included as a validator of the experiences offered as demonstrating competence. This has resource implications but it seems the professional bodies currently support this work, both in pre- and post-registration situations. With that endorsement, then maybe the resource issue will be adequately addressed. However, the cynical may still have reservations as the impact of contracting for services makes securing educational resources difficult. The resource issue notwithstanding the preparation of mentors is key. Certainly in the first instance mentors have no formal experience of reflective learning and associated assessment strategies. Understandably anxieties about performance and expectations run high if no support and feedback are available for mentors. Encouragement to engage in written validation within the learning contract is vital though some mentors remain hesitant about doing so for fear of inadvertently exposing their practice to critical scrutiny. Fostering of an open supportive learning environment is essential, and is addressed elsewhere in the book.

Challenge for practice/practitioners

The challenge for practitioners is two-fold. Firstly the effect of professional judgment in relation to one's own practice, be it the result of personal scrutiny within one's own learning or via the exposure of your own practice to a student. Secondly the imperative for changing or developing practice which is brought to the practitioner's attention. This is particularly challenging when poor practice, if not a disciplinary offence, comes very close to breaking the code of professional conduct. In such situations the episode may be included in a learning contract and indeed the student may have made good use of a potentially negative experience, turning it around and identifying what to do rather than what not to do. As the teacher involved how do you handle this? Can you use the evidence within a contract as part of a challenge to change practice, even taking it so far as to be evidence within a disciplinary situation in the extreme case? Our experience so far shies away from using learning contract evidence in any formal disciplinary way. The contract is the student's property and cannot be used out of context without their permission. However 'whistle blowing' is a key concern in nursing and on a more informal footing learning contract evidence can be shown to ward sisters and practitioners in the form of feedback – positive *and* negative – 'this is how your ward's assessment is or isn't documented – what do you think?' This again must be with the student's permission but it is often, if handled sensitively, good use of unbiased comment.

Conclusions

Experience so far suggests we have developed an effective tool for assessing reflective learning. Modification of the tool has taken place in the light of difficulties encountered. However the fundamental principle of assessing the process of learning as well as the outcome has been adhered to. The grading process clearly focuses on the reflection and therefore has to address the thinking underlying practice. The achievement of competency assures the outcome measure.

A key factor determining the success of assessing reflective learning is the mentor. Preparation and support of individuals who take on the role are vital. Preparation, so the uncertainty of using an unfamiliar learning process can be addressed. Soon we will be in a position where mentors will have personal experience of contracts to draw on when helping students get to grips with the owners. The placement will provide positive support as mentors gain confidence in identifying learning opportunities in their clinical area, recognizing students in difficulty and refining their expectations of student performance with students on a course so different from some of their own experiences. The clinical presence of nurse education in the form of lecturer-practitioners is significant in achieving this.

The assessment tool is in some ways still in its infancy and further development and formal evaluation is required. However we feel it has its place in the range of assessment strategies available for nurse educators.

References

Alexander, M. (1983) *Learning to Nurse: Integrating Theory & Practice.* Churchill Livingstone, London.

Benner, P. (1984) *From Novice to Expert. Excellence & Power in Clinical Nursing Practice.* Addison-Wesley, California.

Bevis, E.O. (1978) *Curriculum Building in Nursing: A Process.* 2nd edition. C.V. Mosby, St. Louis.

Bines, H. & Watson, D. (1992) *Developing Professional Education.* The Society for Research into Higher Education and Open University Press, Buckingham.

Binnie, A. & Titchen, A. (1993) *Developing Professional Practice in a Medical Unit.* National Institute of Nursing, Oxford.

Boud, D., Keogh, R. & Walker, D. (1985) *Reflections: Turning Experience into Learning,* Kogan Page, London.

Bradley, J. & Edinburg, M.A. (1990) *Communication in the Nursing Context.* Appleton & Large, East Norwalk.

Brykczynki, K. (1989) An interpretive study describing the clinical judgment of nurse practitioners. *Scholarly Inquiry for Nursing Practice*, **3**, (2), 75–104.

Carper, B. (1978) Fundamental patterns of knowing. *Advances in Nursing Science*, **1**, 13–23.

Darbyshire, P., Stewart, B., Jamieson, E. & Tongue, C. (1990) New domains in nursing. *Nursing Times*, **86**, 27 July, 73–5.

Dearmun, A. (1993) Reflections of the lecturer practitioner role. *Paediatric Nursing*, **5** (1), 26–8.

Goodman, J. (1984) Reflection & teacher education: A case study & theoretical analysis. *Interchanges*, **15**, 39–25.

Hepworth, S. (1989) Professional judgement & nurse education. *Nurse Education Today*, **9**, 408–12.

Jarvis, P. (1992) Reflective practice & nursing. *Nurse Education Today*, **12**, 174–81.

Lawler, J. (1991) *Behind the Screens. Nursing Comology, the Problem of the Body.* Churchill Livingstone, Melbourne.

Lathlean, J. (1992) The contribution of lecturer-practitioners to theory and practice in nursing, *Journal of Clinical Nursing*, **1**, 237–42.

Long, P. (1976) Judging & reporting on student nurses' clinical performance. *International Journal of Nursing Studies*, **13**, 115–21.

Mezirow, J. (1981) A critical theory of adult learning & education. *Adult Education*, **32**, 1, 3–24.

Newell, R. (1992) Anxiety, accuracy & reflection: the limits of professional development. *Journal of Advanced Nursing*, **17**, 1326–33.

Oxford Polytechnic (1986) Course document – BA Nursing and Midwifery Programme. Oxford Polytechnic, Oxford.

Oxford Polytechnic (1989) Course document Vol 1 The Institutions and Course Dept. Nursing, Midwifery and Health Visiting. Oxford Polytechnic, Oxford.

UKCC (1983) *Nurses & Midwives Rules* United Kingdom Central Council for Nursing, Midwifery & Health Visiting, London.

UKCC (1986) Project 2000 – A new preparation for practice. United Kingdom, Central Council for Nursing, Midwifery & Health Visiting.

UKCC (1990) *The report of the post-registration education & practice project.* United Kingdom Central Council for Nursing, Midwifery & Health Visiting.

Further reading

Akinsanya, J. (1990) The reflective practitioner – is help at hand? *Nursing Standard*, **4**, 20, 33–4.

Ashworth, P. & Morrison, D. (1991) Problems of competence-based nurse education. *Nurse Education Today*, **11**, 256–60.

Benner, P. (1984) *From Novice to Expert Excellence & Power in Clinical Nursing Practice.* Addison-Wesley, California.

Burns, S. (1992) The stuff nightmares are made of, or a useful way to learn nursing? *Teaching News* EMU/Oxford Brookes University, **32**, 18–20.

Burns, S. (1992) Grading practice. *Nursing Times,* **88**, 1, 40–2.

Champion, R. (1988) Competent Nurse? Reflective practitioner paper presented at International Conference on Nursing Education, Cardiff.

Champion, R. (1991) Professional collaboration: The lecturer practitioner role. In *Developing Professional Education.* Ed. H. Bines. Society for Research into Higher Education & Open University, Press, Buckingham.

Clarke, M. (1986) Action & reflection: practice & theory in nursing. *Journal of Advanced Nursing,* **22**, 3–11.

George, P. (1986) The nurse as a reflective practitioner. Unpublished paper: Dept. of Social Studies, Oxford Polytechnic, Oxford.

Girot, E. (1993) Assessment of competence in clinical practice: a phenomenological approach. *Journal of Advanced Nursing,* **18**, 114–19.

Lawton, D. (1981) Curriculum Evaluation in *The Study of the Curriculum.* (ed. P. Gordon). Batsford, London.

Van Manem, M. (1977) Linking ways of knowing with ways of being practical. *Curriculum Enquiry,* **6** (3), 205–28.

Chapter 3
The Mentor's Experience – A Personal Perspective

Introduction

'Brigid uses her ability to challenge and support to great effect here...'

Jan, a student, commenting on me, her mentor.

This was solicited feedback from one student commenting on one specific instance. It is not very often that one receives such direct feedback! It is about one interaction which worked to promote reflection: not all do. Somehow though, through giving attention to the process of reflection, interactions which do not appear productive can be viewed as integral to the experience of ongoing learning. I have found that identifying the strategies which are conducive to learning for individuals makes a difference. Through my experience of using strategies with undergraduate nursing students I aim to offer insight into a mentor's role in promoting and managing reflection.

This chapter is informed from a personal perspective and from educational theory. As a practitioner I found that the role of a mentor was poorly defined, and consequently criticized, by the majority of available literature within nursing education. My own experience has enabled me to respond to some of the criticisms to outline a role that exists and appears to function. For me, offering a flexible and unique balance between strategies of challenge and support for the students is central to being a mentor. Such a skill is complex and involves a high degree of self-awareness. Because of this the needs of the role itself also require consideration if it is to be developed and sustained.

The reflective mentor

Page 5 of The Mentor Handbook (Oxford Polytechnic, 1990) defines a mentor as:

'An experienced, competent practitioner in a clinical area who will work with (the student) on a one-to-one, day-to-day basis.'

In supporting a learner to develop and manage reflection, the mentor must have a grasp not only of clinical practice but also of reflection. Reflection is a process of reviewing an experience of practice in order to describe, analyse, evaluate and so inform learning about practice. In contrast to the vision of quiet contemplation that the word used to create for me there is an active element to reflection. The activity which occurs in reflection involves moving beyond the experience as illustrated by the reflective cycle (Gibbs, 1988) see Fig 3.2. The starting point for the cycle occurs when one questions why an outcome has occurred (Jarvis, 1992). Such a question may arise from a feeling of discomfort (Boyd & Fales, 1983), or from a dramatic event. It is often the latter that novice students focus on. However it is important to recognize that we need to examine when we feel we have been effective and those activities which we take for granted to avoid habitualising our practice (Berger & Luckmann, 1967).

As a mentor who is also a practitioner there is an issue of consciousness of self effect. My own use of reflection to learn from, inform and transform my practice proved valuable in this respect. However I should not assume this is so for other practitioners. Powell (1989) wrote of how the practitioners in her small study had little insight into their actions; they did have knowledge informing them, but could not access or articulate it. Reflecting upon my own development of reflection, environmental factors such as my colleagues' views, have had an important role. My understanding is that Powell's practitioners were previously unexposed to an atmosphere where reflection was promoted. This could be an important consideration, given the potential of reflective practice.

Using reflection can access our 'theories in use' (Powell, 1989), so enabling others to learn. In this way, the risks of taking practice for granted has the potential to be reduced. For example, examining a departure from an unconscious routine in response to an individual's need. Often insight can be gained as to what influenced the action. Thus what we do, our 'artistry' (Schön, 1985), can be explored and shared. In recognizing the role of reflection in this, its skill is relevant for both the student and mentor.

In theory it may be possible to promote reflection without insight into the process but I suspect, from personal experience, that a vital element of congruence is lost. After I had been attempting to reflect by keeping a diary for over a year, a chance conversation revealed to me that for the first time I was conversing with someone who advocated reflection and actually practised it themselves! That a mentor should find some way of developing their reflective thinking is therefore, I believe, conducive to the process. I felt that my skills enabled me to be a credible and insightful role model, less threatened by reflective questioning and in a better position to be an effective validator of the students' contracts (as explored in Chapter 2).

Strategies to promote reflection

Nurse education has increasingly relied upon ideas of adult education (Burnard, 1990); the focus being on learning from experience and the ethos of self direction and responsibility on the part of the student. As I have identified reflection is more than describing experience, indeed in referring to the work of Nevitt Sandford on self reflection, Daloz asserted that it is:

> only by bringing our changes into conscious awareness that we can be assured they will stay put.

> (Daloz, 1986, p. 213)

It is in the involvement of guiding students through such transitions that Daloz feels mentors are vital. This is similar to Schön's (1985) concept of a 'coach'. Burnard (1990) however has doubts about such a close relationship, given the aims of adult education. He argues that rather than encouraging autonomy the mentor is more likely to foster dependence and conformity. It is the recognition of such a danger, and an awareness that adults often vary in their individual learning styles, that influence my consideration of strategies that mentors can use.

The work of Daloz (1986) on what it is that mentors do offers a useful insight. He suggests three main areas of mentor work: *supporting*, *challenging* and *providing vision*. Challenge and support are seen as mutually dependent and their relationship is envisaged in Fig. 3.1. What is important for the mentor to know and recognize is that: 'What is support for one person may be challenge for another' (Daloz, 1986, p. 213). I suspect that it is only when there is a closeness between mentor and student that the mentor will be able to sense which is which and the student will feel able to attempt to articulate this. Indeed Brookfield (1987) talks of how important creating an atmosphere of trust is before one can start to question critically. With this need in mind I want to give attention to the particular elements raised by Daloz (1986). As they are often context specific what I intend to offer are practical examples of instances which were supportive, challenging or which provided vision.

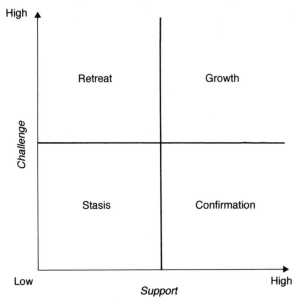

Fig. 3.1 The mutually dependent relationships in mentoring (after Daloz, L.A. (1986) *Effective Teaching and Mentoring: Realizing the Transformation Power of Adult Learning Experiences*, figure on p. 214, Jossey-Bass, Inc, Publishers.)

Supporting

One of the strategies I have found helpful for some students is offering them feedback along the lines of *perceived strengths* and *areas to work on*. This is in addition to their self assessment and reflects the feeling that positive feedback should come first (Northedge, 1990) and will promote the student's self concept. It has been my experience that students really value constructive feedback which offers them insight into why something is or is not effective. There is an issue of developing their own ability to do so but it is also related to experiencing it from others.

In one such feedback session with a student, Jan, I cautiously suggested that from observation I felt that she was unsure about using the ward telephone. This appeared to enable her to discuss how she felt afraid and consequently avoided being involved with its use, particularly when speaking to relatives. Given her response and her indication that it was an area she wanted to address we took it further.

After establishing how she felt we explored what might have contributed to these feelings. Jan identified an experience as a relative in which she had been offered scant information. This led her to want to offer more than the bare minimum yet she recognized that she might not know the patient or relatives well enough, or not feel in a position to take that responsibility. From this I gently probed to elicit what was strong and what was weak about such a position. From this she could see that whilst it was a skill she did not yet have, her awareness of this deficit was vital as it prevented her from operating dangerously! From my feedback I was able to affirm how effective I generally found her communication skills with clients to be and why. We then explored the similarities and differences of communicating on the phone to doing so directly with clients. From this we formed a plan of action which involved:

(1) Joint reflection on how I handled particular phone calls.
(2) Answering all incoming calls to the ward when she was available and directing them to the person concerned.
(3) Jan to note her level of discomfort when admitting that she did not know something but would find someone who did.

This plan was then reviewed at a later date and revised according to Jan's feeling of progress and need. What I was offering were probes to the process of reflection. I find constantly referring to the reflective cycle (Gibbs, 1988) (Fig. 3.2) very helpful with some students. That I was successful in this instance was in part due to the sense of awareness I had of who and where Jan was. For instance some students may need to concentrate on unpicking what is actually happening in a situation. As

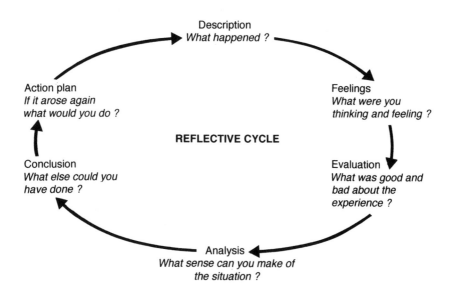

Fig 3.2   The reflective cycle (from Gibbs, 1988).

both Schön (1985) and Powell (1989) recognized, awareness of the experience and an ability to describe it are difficult though essential skills. The joint exploration of the cycle enables the student to identify where they are in terms of their reflection, and reduces the risk of assumptions or misdiagnosis on the part of the mentor. This is another way to increase one's awareness as a mentor and so aids me to ascertain what and how I know; or find an alternative route if I am wrong, which I can be!

Although the process of identifying and addressing need within the reflective cycle can be slow, to leap stages may inhibit learning (Brookfield, 1987) or not equip mentees to transfer the process to other situations. I have experienced the temptation, either on my or the student's part, to go for a 'quick fix' rather than see the development of reflection in the context of ongoing need. Given this proviso I feel that the exemplar demonstrates some of what Daloz (1986) outlines as being skills of supporting:

- Listening
- Providing structure
- Expressing positive expectations
- Serving as an advocate
- Sharing ourselves
- Making it special

Such skills also apply not only to the development of reflection but also its management. As the students use reflection to evidence their learning (as shown in Chapter 2) the issue of how to handle it is important. Often the students find themselves in difficulties as they polarize around one of two extreme positions:

torrent of examples 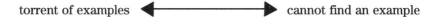 cannot find an example

Often it is a question of learning to 'cash in' on experiences. Whilst this may sound mercenary I find it also promotes a richness of reflection in which one experience can be unpacked to expose so much. This has implications for promoting transferable skills and enabling the focus of reflection to move beyond the self (Goodman, 1984).

Throughout such relationships the mentor needs to bear in mind the risk of overidentification with the student or being carried away in the excitement of discovery. I have found that it is all too easy to presume that just because I can analyse what is happening and see the potential, that the mentee will. To take over could create dependency but is more likely to inhibit learning for the student. There is also the risk that it will blind the mentor to the student's insights which can be equally valid. Awareness of this as a potential risk is vital. I find a way to attempt to avoid this is to suspend belief or notions of a fixed outcome (the outcome can later be matched to the required outcome of competencies and aims). This offers a genuineness in the probing questions such as 'what is happening here?' and 'where does that take you?' that feels helpful. In this way the process of reflection is the mentee's yet the mentor can share in promoting it.

From the exemplar and my cautions it becomes clear that support is not offered in isolation. For instance if I had not taken the risk to gently challenge Jan about the use of the phone the opportunity for support and guidance in addressing it might have been lost. And so within the atmosphere of support I also consider challenge.

Challenging

An instance where challenge was needed was in a relationship involving another student, Ruth. Initially Ruth appeared very quiet and almost timid and much of what I offered was in terms of support. One of Ruth's aims was to develop the skills of cleaning and dressing a wound. I was concerned at her concentration on the task as it did not reflect the holistic nature of the intended learning, though in remembering myself as a student nurse could understand it. After she had watched me doing a dressing several times for a client called Mary, and had got to know Mary, I suggested that Ruth asked Mary if she could perform the dressing. This she did, Mary agreed and with me as a supportive onlooker Ruth did the dressing to her own and Mary's satisfaction.

Following this Ruth expressed her sense of achievement at the successful completion of the task. Whilst I reinforced this I felt that now was the time to take this further. I asked Ruth why the dressing had been successful. She found this difficult to answer except in technical terms. I posed two scenarios in which (1) she was to perform the dressing on a patient she did not know and (2) she was a patient who received fragmented care from different nurses, including a nurse she did not know, to do her dressing. Through this exploration Ruth was able to identify that it had been her relationship with Mary which had been the most significant factor in the successful dressing performance.

A second example is one which occurred with Jan. As the shift progressed it was obvious that Jan had a considerable workload and was tired. Mid-shift she mentioned how she had been distracted from her work the night before and needed to do more before a session on the computer the following day. She then suggested missing the next day's early shift which we had negotiated to work. Internally my reactions were:

- Sympathy to her plight. Jan was generally well organized and ahead with her work (knowing her helped).
- I knew that it was not an easy thing for her to suggest and I did not want to appear inflexible.
- I felt strongly that although she was supernumerary at present, when she qualified she would need to have a work ethos to fulfil her commitment.

My response to Jan was to say 'OK, if that really has to be' but I then asked what she would do if she was working in employment. Jan admitted that she could not have that choice then. In recognizing this awareness I offered a flexible response of going early that night in order to be able to come in the next morning. As it was she stayed working in the coffee room from 7 PM until I left and achieved what she wanted to do whilst still remaining near the clinical environment. Jan's own comment on the situation was:

> 'A compromise was achieved and through Brigid I was made aware of my supernumerary status and its potential for misuse.'

In examining these examples there are direct issues of challenging involved. In his work on promoting critical thinking Brookfield (1987) defines it as:

(1) Identifying and challenging assumptions.
(2) Imagining and exploring alternatives.

Daloz (1986) writes of ways of enabling the students to grow through working to close the distance in the relationship that the mentor deliberately creates. He discusses:

- Setting tasks
- Heating up dichotomies
- Setting high standards
- Constructing hypotheses
- Engaging in discussions

Indeed these skills are involved in what I have recounted. However there are also more factors involved:

(1) *The timing of the challenge.* This involves not just the immediate context; that is, is it a good or a bad time, but also that within the relationship. Brookfield (1987) talks of earning the right to challenge which involves trust building as explored earlier.

(2) *A sense of congruency.* What is being asked of the mentee is nothing that the mentor would not ask of themselves. For example for the mentor to be known as a nurse who asks her-/himself, 'what if?', and articulates their own standards and goals.

(3) *The skill of risk taking.* From personal reflection this involves the consistency of the relationship and how it has developed, the recognition of opportunities, knowing the student's aims and trusting your own judgment.

(4) *The way it is done.* Again I return to the issue of support. One of the concepts I found most challenging was that of challenging students! Indeed I focused on it in my own reflection. One of the strong factors that came through in my exploration was that it is closely related to giving positive feedback. The issues are related because both involve specificity about either what is effective (Gray & Gerrard, 1977) or the challenge being set. Further both flourish if the two key elements of support and challenge are present. Again the fine balance and interrelationship between the two elements, as seen in Daloz's Diagram (Fig. 3.1), are invoked.

Providing vision

Daloz (1986, p. 230) describes vision as:

'The context that hosts both support and challenge in the service of transformation.'

This involves issues of reflective attitudes (Goodman, 1984) and the belief in the juxtaposition of the other two key elements of the mentor's role, those of challenge and support. Most importantly vision is a metaphor for greater understanding. Whilst this may involve role modelling it needs to move beyond it. The mentor is only effective if the object of inspiration is nursing, not just the mentor. This is where the model in which a student has multiple sequential mentors throughout her or his course can have advantages. In the same way that each client is unique so is each nurse and her/his vision of nursing.

There is also an analogy of 'offering a map' (Daloz, 1986) which is similar to the concept of being a 'skilled companion' as Campbell (1984) names the nurse in her/his role with clients. The issue is that of enabling a journey. The mentor/nurse has a clearer idea of the terrain yet it is the mentee/client who should be the determinant of the destination. The skill involved is in knowing the type of companionship to offer in each role. That will depend on the mentee or the client. The mentor can not necessarily avoid the pitfalls inherent in such journeys. Rather the mentor can enable the mentee to:

'know better when she is in one – and thus take fuller advantage of the unique opportunities that most pitfalls offer.'

(Daloz 1986 p. 208)

Whilst exploring my own experiences of being a mentor and drawing from them key elements of the role I found it interesting to consider how that role is defined and perceived by others.

Being a mentor

The term mentor appears to be a diversely used one with little clarity or unity of definition (Morle (1990), Burnard (1990)). The contexts of use encompass the business world (Levinson *et al.*, 1978), higher education (Daloz, 1986), nurses' careers (Darling (1984), Fields (1991)) and nurse education (Burnard (1990), Morle (1990), Donovan (1990)). In developing a definition of a mentor to articulate the role as I experienced it, on the undergraduate nursing degree programme at Oxford Brookes University, I found it enlightening to examine the disparity of views.

Historically the term mentor originates from Homer's *Odyssey*. Upon setting off on his travels Odysseus entrusts his friend Mentor to take care of his son. The concepts of protection, support, enablement and learning appear in envisaging the guidance through role transition. From the literature the influence of the utilisation of mentorship in the business world of the USA is considerable. In this context it is used to describe someone who is at least a role model and more likely to be actively influential in the development of the mentee's career. Even within nursing this role has been related to career development of great nurses, for example Florence Nightingale (Fields, 1991).

The form of the mentor in career development is often seen as involving an older, wiser person who protects and sponsors the mentee. The relationship is not prescribed, rather chosen, and often involves emotional ties (Donovan, 1990). There is recognition that the time span involved is often a matter of years and has a recognizable life cycle (Darling, 1984).

The incorporation of the concept of mentorship within nurse education occurred with the encouragement of the English National Board (ENB, 1988). However as Morle (1990) and Burnard (1990) identify, there was little in the way of guidance as to what the role involved. The definition offered little more other than that the mentor be a first level nurse (ENB, 1988). Obviously there could be advantages to a uniform definition such as avoiding ambiguity and offering a prescription. However Daloz (1986) believes that the role and persona of a mentor will vary from situation to situation. Certainly my experience supports this and whilst I appreciated guidance, prescription from an agent external to the course could have been restrictive. With these considerations in mind I offer a role outline specific to the Oxford undergraduate nursing degree.

In The Mentor Handbook (Oxford Polytechnic, 1990) mentor activities are outlined as follows:

> The mentor is responsible for guiding the students' learning in the clinical area by:
>
> - Initially being with the student on days of the clinical placement.
> - Contracting; encouraging the student to self assess and identify objectives to be met during the placement ensuring that such objectives are relevant to their previous experiences and relevant to the competencies that are to be achieved in the module.
> - Discussing and agreeing the resources and strategies required for their learning.
> - Planning the learning experiences so that the modular competencies can be achieved.
> - Encouraging self assessment by the student and assessing yourself the learning outcomes, ensuring there is adequate evidence to support both the student's assessment and yours of his/her achievement.
> - Identifying and ensuring opportunities are made for the student to reflect on their experiences; initially this is envisaged happening at the end of each shift.
> - Encouraging the student's recording of their experiences as soon as possible after the event by recording in their personal log/diary.
> - Using your lecturer-practitioner and the student's personal tutor for advice or information as necessary.

From this it can be seen that the role is one which Donovan refers to as 'restricted mentoring'. In this the emphasis is on a short term interaction (four to ten weeks) concentrating on the educational needs of the student; in this case the learning contract to demonstrate clinical competence (as discussed in Chapter 2). The mentor is a first level clinical nurse (ENB, 1988) and the relationship is focused and intense (Fields,

1991) due to the nature of working together. Bracken & Davis (1989) raise the potential difficulty of the mentors having to make themselves available. However in my experience students, in accordance with the course philosophy, are expected to fit in with their mentors' times off duty. With the exception of extensive night duty or holiday this is not unrealistic and it is in the student's interest to ensure that this is achieved.

The mentor is more than a role model. Peutz (1988) cited in Donovan (1990) views role modelling as having characteristics which could be considered passive. This is particularly a risk as behaviours may be adopted without understanding the underlying principles or the reasons for the behaviour. In the mentor role I am defining, there is an active element implied in the activities outlined. Although there is a natural concern for the outcome (the learning contract which will be assessed) much of the role focuses on the process; developing and managing reflection. It is only by exploring what it means to be a reflective mentor and some of the strategies available that insight as to *how* the activities on the list can be gained.

From the experiences I have outlined in the chapter, the relationship I have described is often a close one. Indeed in rejecting Burnard's (1990) suggestion that a more detached relationship would serve the purpose better, I feel that it is the development of trust and getting to know each other that can provide an effective foundation.

Forming the relationship

There have been criticisms of the mentor/mentee relationship with regard to the short length of time span afforded to it (Donovan (1990), Barlow (1991)) and the lack of choice in the relationship (Bracken & Davis, 1989). In counteracting such criticisms I find the parallel of the development of a trusting and effective nurse/patient relationship strong. Such a relationship may occur within the space of hours and rarely has a degree of choice in it. The key factors of this relationship building are ones of intent, commitment and atmosphere of purpose (Meutzel, 1988). Although recognizing that the mentor/mentee relationship is different to the nurse/patient one in scope and aim, it is useful for the mentor to build on the skills she or he already possesses as a relationship builder.

Schön (1985) writes of needing a setting of low risk for the student to practise in. Whilst this could be interpreted as a purely physical environment (such as the clinical room in a School of Nursing), within the real world of practice in which students find themselves it is offered in supernumerary status and the relationship of the students with their mentors. Both Daloz (1986) and Brookfield (1987) refer to the creation of trust as a necessary starting point.

Upon meeting the mentee I try to create an atmosphere of trust and establish mutual expectations. How this occurs is very dependent on the individual students and how I'm feeling and as ever the degree of my self awareness is important. For example I may have to tone down my zeal or compensate for fatigue, these being two regular attributes of my mode of work! I invite them to tell me how they have previously worked (clinically and with regard to their learning contracts) and to articulate if they can, their preferred learning style. It is by this means that I attempt to establish what is supportive or challenging for them. For example, one student preferred negotiated and reviewed short term goals whereas another felt that this was intrusive and wanted to go it alone for longer. A mentor can not promise to be all things to all students, however they can be aware of needs and adopt their style in a way that feels congruent to them.

Whilst establishing the mentees' needs it is important that an element of reciprocity occurs. I outline what I have to offer to the mentees; my needs and my expectations of them. This may involve some small personal disclosures to illustrate my human side and certainly indicates areas of perceived weaknesses such as a tendency to expect too much too soon. There is a danger that disclosure may inhibit the mentee or reduce confidence in the mentor. However the projection of credibility and willingness to share have generally felt effective to me.

Whilst the aim of the relationship is to support and manage reflection there has to be an element of congruence throughout the relationship. Reflection is not something one should switch on to as a discrete entity. In his study on working towards a theory of reflection, Goodman (1984) turned to the work of Dewey and Van Manen to offer three mutually dependent elements:

- The focus of reflection
- The process of reflection
- Attitudes to reflection

In clarifying what constitutes reflective attitudes, Goodman (1984) discusses:

(1) *open mindedness* in which things are not taken for granted, and self questioning is promoted.
(2) *responsibility* to make sense of diverse ideas and to move beyond questions of immediate utility.
(3) *wholeheartedness* in which self esteem and commitment are seen as important and enabling in risk taking.

With this view of reflective attitudes and the need for congruency, I find it helps to extend the relationship formation to the clarification of practical roles. This is particularly important as the students are supernumerary. I attempt to clarify the commitment I expect; to me, our patients and the nursing team. In exploring their role with respect to me, I outline a continuum I find most students move along, the pace varying according to their experience and developmental rate:

The continuum of the developing roles of the mentee

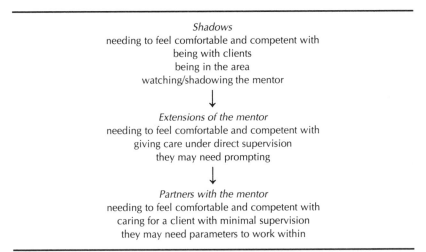

The articulation of expectations does not guarantee a smooth journey, but usually promotes an atmosphere in which problems on either side can be addressed. There also needs to be recognition of a realistic pacing of the journey. As Vaughan & FitzGerald (1992) observed with regard to reflection:

> 'Indeed to try to achieve such a level of enquiry all the time in everyday practice would be utterly exhausting and cumbersome and in itself might constrain creativity.'

(p. 145)

The mentor's needs

The role of mentor articulated in this chapter is skilled and involves commitment and energy on the part of the practitioner. It is therefore appropriate to consider how the mentor develops and sustains her/his self. There are several categories of need: *preparation, support* and *reward.*

Preparation

Nurse registration education has until now offered little formal experience in the skills of facilitating learning. That is not to say that practitioners will not have developed them, but to note that it cannot be assumed. The practitioner who is to become a mentor needs to have several requisites:

- To want to
- Be comfortable and competent in their present role
- Feel open to learning themselves
- Have an awareness of the richness of practice and to value it.

Some have suggested formal qualifications as a basis for becoming a mentor, for example the ENB 998 (Morle (1990), Bracken & Davis (1989)). The acceptability of such courses depends on the focus and depth of their scope and thus needs exploring. These may have a role but it is perhaps an ability to learn rather than to teach that has the greater influence (Schön, 1985). Personally it has been the development of my own *reflective skills* within the support of a Certificate in Further Education that has been particularly useful.

Certainly some formal preparation specific to the role of mentor, both at the outset and then as a development tool, is essential. This needs to address two factors, the interpersonal skills role and the organisational role. The former should consider reflection and the strategies I outline. The latter needs to encompass the mentees' course, their goals and what is expected of them. My preparation involved a session in which I reflected on people who had been significant in my development and the skills they had. A mentee recently suggested that examining our own learning styles and having an awareness of how individuals differ would be useful. In my preparation an invitation for us to construct our own learning contracts to use to focus our early reflections generated the following personal objectives:

(1) To balance my roles as a patient care giver, senior nurse on a shift and mentor.
(2) To feel a competence and ease in challenging students when necessary.

My needs of preparation continued to be met through close contact with the lecturer-practitioner who was responsible for my mentor preparation and the students' clinical placements. With the lecturer-practitioner I was able to have a supervisory relationship (as discussed in Chapter 8) in which I could reflect on my experience as a mentor in order to develop my skills. The integrated nature of the role of lecturer-practitioner, who has close contact with both parties in the clinical setting, therefore promotes the development of mentors by ensuring that their needs are given continued attention.

Support for the mentor

Support can be offered formally through those involved in the course, either the lecturer-practitioners or mentor support groups. I experienced supervision through the process of appraisal with my line manager. Being in supervision as a practitioner (as discussed in Chapter 8) offers further aid particularly in learning to become self reflective. Often the question 'how do you know when you've been effective?' is asked of practitioners, and mentors should not be exempt. Through reflection and reception of the appropriate balance of support and challenge I can attempt to ascertain my effectiveness. It can sometimes be enticing to rely on feelings of being liked as testimony to effect. As Brookfield (1987) highlights in cautioning against this, some learning involves frustration and so possible discomfort. Finding mechanisms to discern these factors and to accommodate them whilst retaining self esteem can be facilitated through supervision.

The organizations, both of practice and education, need to recognize and value the role of mentor. Although they are not able to reward it materially, values can be transmitted through behaviour and effect self esteem and so the commitment of those involved. Support from colleagues as they recognise the increased demands on the mentor is invaluable. This does not necessarily involve taking over aspects of the mentor's practice; simply demonstrating an awareness that support could be needed and promoting teamwork is usually sufficient. Another source of support is often the clients, both to the mentees and mentor. I have often been boosted by their interest, tolerance and an attitude that such a role is somehow special.

Reward

I think it is important to ask 'what do I get out of this?' The potential of motivation is one of the vital elements ensuring the success of the role. As registered nurses the development of other nurses is inherent to our role but never before has this been so instrumental and demanding.

From personal and anecdotal evidence, supported by Tongue (1992) there is a strong element of reciprocity in the relationship. Tongue's respondents commented on what they had learnt from their students. This learning encompasses not only new knowledge transmitted from students but increased insight into and an ability to be reflective about what we do as practitioners.

On commenting on how supportive she found the ward environment to be a student responded to my question of 'I wonder what makes it so?' She did this by creating an objective in her learning contract about it. The evidence she provided was a very useful perspective to have for those of us so immersed in it. Additionally in the development of a frequently close relationship there is often a great deal of practical and emotional support from the students which should not be under-estimated. However the degree to which the students are felt to be supportive depends on their approach and the mentor's feeling of comfort in the examination of her/his practice.

Summary

There are limitations to this personal exploration of the role in that there is little other than my own experience to draw on in terms of reality. However this has enabled me to offer elements of a practical model with which to support what I believe is a powerful educational tool. I have highlighted that the instrumental factor in the role of mentor is self awareness. If consideration is given to the preparation and the needs of the role then practitioners can gain a chance to develop themselves and their understanding of nursing. If this is combined with an awareness of learners' individual needs, there is the potential for the ongoing balance of challenge and support to be facilitated in a journey of joint discovery. My journeys have not been without pitfalls, yet the effect of each has been to enhance my understanding of myself and nursing in some way. The fulfilment of also enabling another in their development is a significant reward. The potential benefits of such mutual development indicate that such a role requires further consideration and opportunity in the growth of the professional practitioner.

References

Barlow, S. (1991) Impossible Dream, *Nursing Times*, **87**, 153–4.
Berger, P. & Luckmann, T. (1967) *The Social Construction of Reality*, Penguin, London.

Boyd, E.M. & Fales, A.W. (1983) Reflective learning: Key to learning from experience, *Journal of Humanistic Psychology*, **23**, (2), 99–117.

Bracken, E. & Davis, J. (1989) The implication of mentorship in nursing career development, *Senior Nurse*, **9**, 5, 15–16.

Brookfield, S.D. (1987) *Developing Critical Thinkers*. Open University Press, Milton Keynes.

Burnard, P. (1990) The student experience: adult learning and mentorship revisited, *Nurse Education Today*, **10**, 349–54.

Campbell, A. (1984) *Moderated Love: a Theology of Professional Care*, Society for the Propagation of Christian Knowledge, London.

Daloz, L.A. (1986) *Effective Teaching and Mentoring*, Jossey-Bass Ltd, London.

Darling, L. (1984) Mentor types and life cycles, *The Journal of Nursing Administration*, **14**, 11, 43–4.

Donovan, J. (1990) The concept and role of mentor, *Nurse Education Today*, **10**, 294–8.

ENB Circular 1988/39/APS Institutional and course approval/reapproval process, information required, *Criteria and Guidelines*. English National Board, London.

Fields, W.L. (1991) Mentoring in nursing: a historical approach. *Nursing Outlook*, **39**, 6, 257–61.

Gibbs, G. (1988) *Learning by Doing: A guide to teaching and learning methods*. Further Education Unit, Oxford Polytechnic, Oxford.

Goodman, J. (1984) Reflection and teacher education: A case study and theoretical analysis. *Interchange*, **15**, 3, 9–26.

Gray, W.A. & Gerrard, B.A. (1977) *Learning by Doing: Developing Teaching Skills*. Addison-Wesley, London.

Jarvis, P. (1992) Reflective practice and nursing. *Nurse Education Today*, **12**, 174–81.

Levinson, D. *et al.* (1978) cited in Donovan, J. (1990). The concept and role of mentor, *Nurse Education Today*, **10**, 294–8.

Meutzel, P.A. (1988) Therapeutic Nursing. In Pearson, A. (ed.) (1988) *Primary Nursing*, Croom Helm, London.

Morle, K.M.F. (1990) Mentorship – is it a case of the emperor's new clothes or just a rose by any other name? *Nurse Education Today*, **10**, 66–9.

Northedge, N. (1990) *The Good Study Guide*, Open University Press, Milton Keynes.

Peutz, (1988) cited in Donovan, J. (1990). The concept and role of mentor, *Nurse Education Today*, **10**, 294–8.

Powell, J.H. (1989) The reflective practitioner in nursing, *Journal of Advanced Nursing*, **14**, 824–32.

Schön, D. (1985) *Educating the Reflective Practitioner*, Jossey-Bass, San Francisco.

Tongue, C. (1992) Mentorship: what is it and does it work? unpublished paper given at the Institute of Nursing, Oxford, 22nd October 1992.

Vaughan, B. & Fitzgerald, M. (1992) Caring for the acutely ill, in Vaughan, B. & Robinson, K. (eds.) (1992) *Knowledge for Nursing Practice*, Butterworth Heinemann, Oxford.

Chapter 4
Reflection – A Student's Perspective

Introduction

Are you feeling confounded by reflection and overawed by adult and self-directed learning? This is how we felt on just leaving school and embarking on higher education. As undergraduate student nurses we were facing a new course in a strange place with unfamiliar people and we were expected to start to take responsibility for our own learning through the use of reflection on our professional practice.

The aim of this chapter is to present an insight into the experience of becoming a reflective practitioner through the eyes of two undergraduate nurses beginning a career in nursing. Included in this chapter are several extracts from our learning contracts which are reflective accounts written during the second and third year of the course programme. As a first level pre-registration student the transition into reflective practice can be an arduous one. It will probably be the first time an individual has had the opportunity to examine his or her personal and professional beliefs and knowledge. This experience can be many things: humbling, disturbing, boring, even inspirational. However, it always appears to be a learning experience.

You may believe reflection has little relevance to you as a student. We aim to challenge this assumption through sharing some of our reflective extracts with you and providing appropriate comment on the impact each example has had on our personal and professional development. By engaging with us on this reflective journey we anticipate that you too may begin to see reflection as a valuable part of your development towards providing therapeutic nursing care. This chapter also aims to offer some reassurance to novice reflective practitioners in facing the uncertainty which lies ahead. We believe this chapter furthermore raises important issues for those senior practitioners and educators who support and guide other novice practitioners through the process of reflection.

Our initial difficulties with learning through reflection were augmented by our previous educational experiences. From a didactic, pedagogic approach to teaching and learning at school we encountered something quite different on commencing our nursing education. We were confronted with an open and sharing approach to learning which encouraged us to set and achieve our own learning needs with support and guidance. Instead of 'doing' because we were told to, we were required to take responsibility and have charge of our own learning.

We were encouraged to reflect on our experience, analysing our reactions and feelings towards issues raised in practice. By documenting these reflections in a diary, they would serve as a useful source of information when writing a learning contract. Our level of reflection and competence in practice was assessed using this learning contract, which required us to identify what we wanted to learn, how we would accomplish it, and documentation of examples of reflective analysis from our clinical practice which fulfilled the identified learning objectives. In reality students found that after a day spent in clinical practice, it was often difficult to sit down and document personal reflection, particularly if experiences of the day had been traumatic or challenging. However to record difficult incidents could prove highly therapeutic and rewarding through the development of self awareness.

Initially, reflecting and documenting reflection was harder than anticipated and was often very descriptive; lacking in analysis. Reflective extract 1 demonstrates the descriptive level of the reflection during a student's first placement in practice. It is not well written due to a lack of nursing knowledge and a high level of anxiety about the correct way to make reflection explicit.

Reflective extract 1

'Boy, aged 5, was admitted to hospital as he had been suffering from extremely bad headaches and delirium. He was thought to have meningitis. My knowledge about meningitis was very, very limited so I asked my mentor to explain so I could appreciate the treatment he was receiving.

Meningitis is an infection which is initially found in the blood; for this reason a blood test was taken. It spreads quickly and crosses the blood–brain barrier into the cerebral spinal fluid; for this reason he had a lumbar puncture. The boy was rushed into hospital and was treated immediately; they felt they had caught the spread of infection before it reached the blood–brain barrier. He was given paracetamol to reduce his temperature.

Meningitis can affect the production of anti-diuretic hormone, causing the body to re-absorb most of its water and therefore dilute the body's essential irons and minerals; for this reason he was only allowed fluid via a drip. He was also kept in isolation.'

The reflection is descriptive and shallow containing no analysis or self-awareness. Moreover it is superficial, demonstrating no reflection concerning the nurse's influence on the situation or the influence it had on her. Only the illness the boy was suffering and some of the physical treatments administered were referred to. No research findings were utilized. Furthermore some of the facts stated were incorrect and the rationales given for aspects of his treatment were unsubstantiated. The extract, although poor, is a realistic representation of the level of reflection in the context of the student's lack of experience, of coping strategies and of confidence at this early stage. It is important that initial attempts to reflect, regardless of the standard of this reflection, are rewarded and encouraged with constructive, critical feedback.

At the outset we struggled with the concept of reflection. It seemed so intangible to us. Moving into reflection and higher education felt like learning to swim in deep, cold and unfamiliar waters. Everything was different and unrecognizable. It was difficult to see how one could ever be reflective.

Reflective extract 2

> 'Trying very hard to get down to my learning contract and reflection, I am getting very, very stressed. I don't know what I'm expected to be reflecting on, I cannot see how I can achieve the competencies let alone prove that I have achieved them ... *I want to do well* and I want to be able to assert myself enough so I can *help myself* to do well.'

This reflective extract demonstrates the initial frustration and anxiety the student felt about using reflection and learning contracts. It describes the lack of confidence and self-esteem experienced. The student was aware of her inexperience and of how far she had yet to develop. This was a humbling yet significant realization.

Unlike writing an essay, there are no definitive rules on how to reflect. No one method is universally correct. Without comprehensive guidelines we found writing a learning contract based on our reflections harder than we envisaged. As novice reflectors we sought structure and direction; someone to tell us how to do it. For lecturer-practitioners to have given in to such demands for structure and example, at this stage, might have hindered students in developing individual reflective skills. Yielding such control in your own learning may appear daunting at first. However, the more you utilize it, the more you realize how exciting, creative and challenging it can become.

We soon learnt that self-directed learning in practice was a partnership based on negotiation between student, mentor and lecturer-practitioner. It was important to support and guide rather than reproach and hinder each other as we started our difficult and risky journey. It was through constructive criticism, encouragement and the offer of personal space that the transition into reflective practice could be facilitated.

We began to gain confidence through the support available. This enabled us to develop our own reflective skills; for some students this involved the use of reflective diaries which were often written after each day spent in practice. Others preferred to retain thoughts and reflections in their memory, only writing small notes occasionally, as reminders of the situation. Some students alternatively chose to reflect only during allocated practice times, though most would admit that there were times when it was necessary to take their reflections home with them, preferring to reflect in a different, though familiar environment. Most students have found it beneficial to take time out during practice to reflect informally, with mentors or other practitioners who can facilitate reflection on actual aspects of practice. They can be potent in guiding the students' reflection in other directions and with greater analysis, and in leading them to alternative resources, such as expert practitioners and pertinent research.

Reading a challenging piece of literature can extend our thought processes and help develop and justify the final theory, action or perspective we achieve. Other aids to reflection include close friends who can offer a non-nursing and lay person's perspective. A valuable aid to reflection has been, and still is, the personal time offered through the privileged position of supernumerary status. This, we believe, demonstrates the respect and importance that is placed on time and freedom for reflection.

How and when do you reflect?

There are no set rules on the ideal way to reflect, and you will find that, with experience, you will gradually build up your own framework. It is helpful however, to have an idea of questions you can ask yourself in order to focus your thinking on a situation, eventually incorporating not only reflections on your own actions, but ethical, political and broader social issues that develop for a given experience.

Choose a situation

Ask yourself:

- What was my role in this situation? Did I feel comfortable or uncomfortable? Why?
- What actions did I take? How did I, and others act? Was it appropriate?
- How could I have improved the situation for myself, the patient, my mentor?
- What can I change in future?
- Do I feel as if I have learnt anything new about myself?
- Did I expect anything different to happen? What and why?
- Has it changed my way of thinking in any way?
- What knowledge from theory and research can I apply to this situation?
- What broader issues, for example ethical, political or social, arise from this situation? What do I think about these broader issues?

Reflective extracts 3 and 4 demonstrate the student becoming more analytical and self-aware. The extracts describe two very different situations. However they are similar in that they illustrate the student becoming more reflective about her responsibilities as a nurse and how her actions and knowledge affect those around her.

Reflective extract 3

'I feel that my pharmacological knowledge was greatly lacking when I started on the ward. Because of this limited knowledge I found it helpful to refer to the BNF [British National Formulary] and was constantly gaining knowledge from my mentor and other members of the team.

I have also become more aware of my professional responsibilities – I am accountable and individually responsible to my patients for my decisions and actions. I am only now realizing how serious this is, and admit that at the beginning of the placement I was possibly administering drugs without sufficient thought to my responsibility and accountability. I am required to serve the patients' best interests to the level of my training. I felt at the beginning of my placement that my past experience and training had not equipped me with much knowledge and competence about drugs which I feel has been increased greatly in this placement.

I feel that my future learning should be focusing on specific groups of drugs and individual drugs in each of these groups, not only during my practical placements, but with some more background reading.'

Reflective extract 4

'I found myself in a situation with a client who was under the section of the Mental Health Act, which restricted her freedom to leave the unit. Alice was attempting to leave the unit, she was very determined. I felt very scared and found it hard to reason with her. It was an emotional and physical strain actually to prevent her from leaving. I felt out of my depth. I talked to my mentor about my fear of being hurt and of not being able to stop someone leaving. I would feel responsible if something went wrong as a result of them leaving. I asked my mentor to show me some restraining techniques. The next time I was in this situation with Peter [another patient] I felt more confident and more in control, although I was still fairly scared as I didn't know him or know how he would react.'

These extracts show that we are beginning to examine issues related to us as nurses and how we respond to aspects of care. The feelings described are more personal. There is some attempt to question the knowledge and skills surrounding the care we are offering. Reflection is beginning, tentatively, to be used as a learning process. We have begun to assess what we have achieved and what we still need to achieve. By identifying issues and incidents which are challenging to our beliefs, skills and knowledge, we are able to identify where we need to direct our learning and to set objectives accordingly.

The process of reflection often leads us to a changed perspective of the situation or a different action if the situation recurs. Although we may learn to tackle something in a different way this does not mean we have conquered the dilemma and become an expert; rather we may need to re-examine the issue again at a future date. Reflection does not always offer us solutions, but it does bring clarity and understanding to a situation which might have otherwise remained obstructive to our development. In this way we find that reflection can be inspirational and liberating, as it allows us to understand the profession we are preparing to be a part of.

Initially we found the concept of reflection difficult to grasp, seeing it purely as a time consuming method fulfilling the academic requirements of our course. Reflection has now become established as an integral part of our nursing practice as we try to reflect at a deeper level, not only in our own actions and feelings, but on the wider issues which confront nursing and our professional practice.

Reflective extracts 5, 6 and 7 were written during the third year of the undergraduate course. They present a few of the brushstrokes of the reflective picture created over this time.

Reflective extract 5

'A survey from Riverside Health Authority suggests that "75% of district nurses spend at least a quarter of their time treating leg ulcers" (Poulton, 1991). I would suggest that the same applies to the district nurses I have been working with. I think the statement is incorrect in that the time is not spent simply or solely treating the leg ulcer. To simply "treat an ulcer" is probably ineffective and unhelpful for both patient and nurse. It is obvious in so many of the patients I have met that their needs far exceed the mere physical.

Barry (who is 74 years old) lost his wife last year, he misses her very much. He has suffered with leg ulcers on and off for the past 30 years. They are presently being treated by the district nurses. Each time we have visited him he has been very pleased to see us and talks at length about what he has been doing recently. He always mentions his wife and describes his grief and his loneliness. It is in Barry's interest to continue his leg ulcer problem as it offers him an excuse for company from the district nurses who he gets on so well with. "Loneliness is a precipitating factor in many illnesses and in attention seeking behaviour. It is essential that psychological and social needs are recognised as such and not treated as medical problems." (Wise, 1986)

If as a nurse I misunderstand the need for holistic care and find myself in a situation as described, I could see the patient as irresponsible for not adhering to the treatment I am offering for his leg ulcer. If however I can appreciate that Barry's loneliness is as great a problem as his leg ulcer then I can begin to offer him the sort of care he is looking for. I can avoid the personal frustration by accepting that being an effective practitioner is not merely about healing a leg ulcer, in this case it can also be about healing a broken heart!'

This extract describes the beliefs that nursing is about caring for the whole person and for their needs as the client sees them. This is something that nursing is increasingly embodying. It may appear to the reader to be nothing new. However what is so pertinent is that to develop this theory through personal experience is many times more meaningful than being told it or reading it somewhere in a book.

Reflective extract 6

Larson (1987) (cited in Benner & Wrubel, 1989)) found in a study of 495 nurses that 20% feared making a mistake. They also fear not being able to keep up to date with the knowledge demands. This understandable fear is rendered more stressful because nurses often keep their fear of making a mistake a secret from their colleagues.

The first shifts I spend on X Ward I found difficult, challenging, intimidating and filled with uncertainty. On further reflection I believe these difficulties were related to unexplored and questionable personal and professional expectations of myself. Every week, possibly every shift I learn something new about my beliefs about myself as a nurse; this often means "throwing out the window" some of my existing beliefs. (Many of my ideas about what I am as a nurse have been firmly flung out the window since commencing my nursing education.)

Arriving on the ward I was very aware that this was an oncology ward. I think I began to focus more and more on the fact the patients were dying cancer patients rather than people living with cancer. I was aware of my lack of knowledge regarding treatments for cancer and that I would not be involved in patients' chemotherapy. I felt quite useless. I felt I would fit in better and be more accepted if I could demonstrate impressive knowledge and physical nursing skills. I felt like a novice in the field of experts, even the patients knew more than me. How could I do anything of any worth?

My mood was really low. I felt I couldn't even initiate simple communication with patients. At the time I was working with a patient whose lung cancer rendered him very breathless and greatly restricted in his mobility.

Sometimes when I spoke to him he simply wouldn't respond. Working with him seemed to reinforce my sense of failure. I interpreted his unresponsiveness to me personally and felt useless that I could offer him no advice about his drugs. By focusing on my lack of knowledge of chemotherapy drugs and inability to be involved in their administration I left myself, within my own expectations, in a redundant and useless situation. I wanted the security and certainty of technological and physical aspects of care in this ocean of uncertainty. I couldn't even achieve this.

I decided to leave the ward, have a cry, and partake in some soul searching. I worked through the issues I have discussed and set myself off on a different path with a different destination and a different foundation of belief to see me through. I concluded that I was a novice and that in this situation the patients were the people I needed to learn from. I decided that I would have to let go of my desperate struggle to find acceptability and security, as this was actually causing the opposite effect, I was feeling vulnerable, frustrated and isolated. I needed to start taking some risks, face some uncertainties and allow myself to learn.

'Nursing is intimate and particular. Expert communication helps in understanding the illness and the disease provides unique ways of helping. But there is no way to guarantee the success of caring. Some patients are more accessible and understandable to some nurses than others are. The hallmark of the expert nurse is the recognition of her or his strengths and weaknesses and the ability to shape her or his practice towards strengths.'

(Benner & Wrubel, 1989, p. 385)

Reflective extract 6 is a very revealing piece of reflection and was extremely challenging and difficult to write. The catalyst for this reflection lay in the student's conviction that if she did not face up to her inappropriate and unhelpful beliefs, she would be unable to progress. The personal constructs developed from this experience, have enabled the student to free herself from the guilt of incompetence and enabled her to celebrate and uphold the competence she has.

The student's mentor commented alongside her reflection:

'I think she now realises that nobody knows "everything" but everybody knows "something".'

Reflective extract 7

'Whilst Bill was having a scan I felt very uncomfortable as the radiologist pointed out that Bill had metastases throughout his liver. Considering the seriousness of this diagnosis it felt wrong that I should know more than Bill about his illness. It was a strange experience watching Bill lying in the scanner innocent of the knowledge I had that he was going to die. As we walked back to the ward I dreaded Bill asking me how the scan went. What would I say? Would I lie? Bill didn't ask me anything. I imagine if it was me I would want to know immediately of any result. Possibly Bill didn't want to know or he didn't want to put me in a difficult position or maybe he was just used to being a part of the system and accept passively waiting for a result.

Bill was extremely low during this admission. He was feeling very unwell and was uncertain of both his long and short term prospects. He was unclear whether he was moving wards, or when he was going home, what his diagnosis was and whether he was going to have chemotherapy. Bill was losing control and certainty in his life. Bill went home and was readmitted 3 weeks later. During these 3 weeks he had been told his diagnosis of terminal cancer of the liver.

Bill was like a different man on readmission to the ward. Physically he was walking around and was not as breathless as he had been. He appeared happy (although he would weep at times this was open and seen as constructive grieving). It was as if Bill was taking back control of his life. He talked openly about his death and of the regrets he had and the things he must do before he dies, mainly to take his son to Disney World. It was as if by accepting his death Bill was finding new meaning to his life.

When one's life is threatened you are forced into an exploration of what your life means to you and others and what is and is not important in your life.'

Reflective extracts 5, 6 and 7 need little commentary. They are each recognizable as meaningful, reflective journeys for the student; describing the development of a set of ideas and perspectives on the realities of nursing and caring, and the student's role in those perspectives.

What does reflection mean to us, as students?

- It causes us to make a conscious attempt to identify and study what is happening, and to learn from that (Burnard, 1991).
- It allows us to view situations from different perspectives.
- It acknowledges the student as an individual who retains control by facilitating self-directed learning and enabling us to identify our own particular learning needs.
- Through reflection, not only on successful but unsuccessful actions and the

emotions experienced, we will recognize our strengths and weaknesses, i.e. it facilitates self-analysis and self-evaluation of effectiveness in all situations and encourages personal development through change.
- It fosters responsibility and accountability.
- It allows us to amalgamate appropriate theory with our practice.

Since 1990 we feel that reflection has developed into more than just a learning tool. It has encouraged us to become more aware, questioning the validity of our own and others' actions in relation to care. Our experience of reflection has also equipped us with the necessary knowledge and skills to begin to develop a personal profile of our professional development.

Reality is a messy business, which no text book can truly prepare you for. Nursing is intimate with reality, and reflection offers us the ability to face the real uncertainties which lie ahead. Reflection is futile if the process does not lead to eventual action. The need for reflection to encompass action brings it in touch with reality. In a time when, increasingly, we are expected to justify and evaluate our actions the reflective processes we have developed will equip us with the skills of rationalised and articulate debate to challenge others and defend ourselves and our actions.

Reflection enables us to find clarity and conclusion in the midst of confusion and conflict.

References

Benner, P. & Wrubel, J. (1989) *The Primacy of Caring: Stress and Coping in Health and Illness*, Addison-Wesley, California.

Burnard, P. (1991) Improving through reflection. *Journal of District Nursing*, May, 10–12.

Larson,. (1987) cited in Benner, P. & Wrubel, J. (1989) *The Primacy of Caring: Stress and Coping in Health and Illness*, Addison-Wesley, California.

Poulton, B. (1991) Factors influencing patient compliance. *Nursing Standard Supplement*, **12**, Vol 5, No. 5

Wise, G. (1986) Overcoming loneliness. *Nursing Times*, May 28, 37–42.

Chapter 5
Theories of Reflection for Learning

Introduction

This chapter has been put into the middle of the book intentionally to avoid the impression that theories should necessarily be studied before practice. Whilst intellectual ruminations are interesting and may be helpful, an appreciation of these views is not essential to the nursing student who wants to learn from reflection. Indeed, most of the readers of this chapter will have learnt from their reflections on experience without studying the literature referred to here, and they will almost certainly find their experience useful when considering the following examination of the subject. On the other hand an intellectual enquiry concerning reflection in nursing is necessary for those who recommend, and in some instances dictate, its use.

Despite the fact that the amount of nursing literature concerning reflection is growing, educationalists still dominate the field. Adler (1991, p. 139) writes that rhetoric regarding the reflective practitioner is now so pervasive within the discipline of education that it appears as if critical reflection is favoured and accepted as a dominant discourse. I would suggest that the same emphasis upon reflection as a learning system is happening in the world of nursing, with concurrent effects on the way we research, plan curricula, view sources of knowledge, debate and talk about nursing.

Some contemporary thinkers (Turner (1992), Shapiro (1990)) recommend scepticism in relation to 'grand discourses'. Two reasons for this caution are: that one prevalent discussion simply replaces another; and that the notions associated with the dominant discourse become so influential that alternative views, especially those of the minority, are likely to be silenced. Whilst wary of grand discourses, I as many other nurses, am attracted to the ideas of learning from reflection on and in action or experience (Schön, 1987). I agree with Adler (1991) that the time to review critically what we mean by learning through reflection or the reflective practitioner is more than ripe, in order that this potentially useful perspective can be appreciated in a temperate fashion.

In this chapter I review different views of reflection for learning, concentrating on two in particular. Following this I consider the process of reflective learning, although I am cautious here because from my own lonely experience in the early days of reflecting critically on my nursing practice, and from the frustrated pleas of students for direction, I know that people turn hopefully to the literature for some 'how to' directions. It seems that there is no recipe for how to 'do reflection' but there are plenty of issues worth considering. I believe that the reader will find the other chapters in the book more useful as their descriptions of the experience of learning through reflection may seem more realistically and practically accessible. Penultimately there is a discussion of the attraction that this way of learning has for contemporary nurses, including some notes of caution. Lastly there is a discussion of research and reflection.

Views of reflection for learning

Reflection on and in action and critical inquiry have been chosen for most attention, because they are the perspectives referred to most often when nurses discuss learning through experience (Powell, 1991). They were the ones studied and referred to when the Oxford nursing curriculum was created and established (George (1986), Oxford Brookes University (1988), Champion (1992)).

Of course there are other theoretical views of reflection and these should be acknowledged as legitimate, even if they are not particularly suited to the way we wish to learn the craft of nursing. For instance Descartes (1984, p. 127), the modern proponent of reductionism, exemplified by the infamous mind body split, immortalized the idea of the power of thought in his maxim 'I am thinking therefore I exist'. As a significant figure in the development of modern empirical science his notion of learning through reflection is not what most of the current nursing educationalists have in mind when they refer to 'the reflective practitioner'. In a literature search Adler (1991, p. 139) found several different meanings ascribed to reflection and she argued that there is a pressing need for clarification of perspective to avoid quite understandable confusion.

For instance Benner (1984) and Benner & Wrubel (1989) in their endeavour to uncover the concepts of expert nursing and caring ask nurses to reflect and recount their experiences. However their main focus, quite legitimately as phenomenologists, is upon discovering the essence of the phenomenon rather than the narrator's formal learning. It may be that the recounting of the experience leads the narrator to new understandings and that educationalists may use the work in this manner. However, in this instance, phenomenology is a research methodology not a learning technique. Learning from reflection involves students critically analysing and interpreting their own work, albeit with help in some cases from a mentor, preceptor or coach.

Reflection is an idea used in ordinary and educational life. On the one hand reflection is a loosely used concept, easily assimilated into spontaneous everyday action, and on the other hand it can become a complex, difficult to explain and perplexing phenomenon. The straightforward definition of the verb reflect is 'to cast back (light, heat, etc.), to give back or show an image of; to think carefully, meditate on'. (*The Macquarie Dictionary*, 1991.) However philosophical inquiry regarding the nature of human knowledge (epistemology) leads the investigator to alternative and more elaborate conceptions of the process of acquiring knowledge from reflection.

A grasp of the epistemological perspective taken personally, collectively as a profession or adopted by others is revelationary because these perspectives show how knowledge is sought, developed, appreciated and indeed why it might deviate from another view (Sater (1988), Robinson & Vaughan (1992)). People's way of pursuing truth affects why and how they reflect, what the outcomes of the process of reflection might be and the language they use to portray it. For example the person who believes in an absolute truth pursued through deductive reasoning will reflect in a logical analytical way in order to make a correct decision and defend the decision using words like 'reliability' and 'generalizability'. This logical deductive reasoning is a form of reflection I appreciate as a perspective held to be useful by many, although one which some may argue is limited by its nature.

In the field of nursing Clarke (1986) wrote one of the earliest papers describing the use of reflection for professional development and based it on John Shotter's theories of the psychology of personal action. Clarke (1986, p. 5) mentions that Shotter aimed to conform to the scientific paradigm. I would suggest that this approach is perceptible in a much later paper by a colleague of Clarke's. Newell (1992, p. 1327) proffers the argument that:

'The issues of bias in forgetting and selection at acquisition suggest that accurate reflection may be either impossible or so fundamentally flawed as to be of little value'.

In the paper Newell uses the language of empirical science and the methods of behavioural psychologists to criticize and solve problems he sees in work that originates from a different epistemological perspective. This other perspective Schön (1987) argues acknowledges and accepts uncertainty and subjective experience as valid. Appreciation of Schön's approach is essential to a critique of his work. The understanding philosophical circumspection can bring to a subject is the reason why a number of the authors, when considering reflection as a learning method, give an epistemological preamble to their work (Mezirow (1981), Schön (1983) and (1987), Carr & Kemmis (1986), Smyth (1986), Street (1988)).

Reflection on and in action

As most of the authors explain, learning by thinking of experience is not a new concept. In modern times Dewey (1933) is usually acknowledged as the first educationalist to write about reflection on experience. Nurses became intrigued by the subject as they developed nursing education in the tertiary sector (Deakin University (1988), Oxford Brookes University (1988)).

There appears to be a particular interest in the work of Schön (1983 and 1987) who describes learning for professional work. Schön devotes considerable space in both books to epistemological arguments regarding the inappropriate dominance of technical rationality in professional education. He describes technical rationality as:

> 'an epistemology of practice derived from positivist philosophy, built into the very foundations of the modern research university. Technical rationality holds that practitioners are instrumental problem solvers who select technical means best suited to particular purposes. Rigorous professional practitioners solve well-informed instrumental problems by applying theory and technique derived from systematic preferably scientific knowledge.
>
> (Schön, 1987, 3–4)

This positivistic stance is suited to solving simple problems in contrived situations, rather than the complex urgent and often surprising problems Schön knows practitioners deal with in practice. Furthermore people taking the technical rational view do not give credit to the practitioners' demonstrated intellectual agility in practice. Schön (1983 and 1987) posits that knowledge is embedded in and demonstrated through the artistry of everyday practice, in clever things done 'on the job' and yet which are typically so difficult to describe linguistically and, to the frustration of positivistic scientists, impossible to control.

Argyris & Schön (1974, 1978) have developed the idea of 'theory in use'. They propose that practitioners choose their actions with due consideration for the particular situation and use theories generated from their repertoire which is made up of experience, education, values, beliefs and past strategies. Often these theories are implicit in sponta- neous behaviour and surface only upon reflection on performance, or when the person is confronted with a problem in practice and has to think deliberately which course of action to take.

Reflection in action is the process whereby the practitioner recognizes a new situation or a problem and thinks about it while still acting. Schön (1987) and Boud & Walker (1991) believe it is possible to encourage reflection in action and improve the practitioner's ability to identify problems in the social milieu (enframe problems) and attend to the relevant surrounding stimuli in order to deal with these problems immediately. Whilst problems are not usually exactly the same as on previous occasions, the skilled practitioner is able to select, re-mix or re- cast responses from previous experiences, when deciding how to solve a problem in practice. It should be noted that knowledge of conventional theories may be part of the practitioner's repertoire and play a part in the reflection in action.

Reflection on action is the retrospective contemplation of practice undertaken in order to uncover the knowledge used in a particular situation, by analysing and interpreting the information recalled. The reflective practitioner may speculate how the situation might have been handled differently and what other knowledge would have been helpful.

This reflective process is far more flexible and realistic than the technical rational approach in which espoused theories, those talked about and taught away from the practice arena, are expected but cannot hope to accommodate all of the complications that arise in practical situations. These espoused theories are rejected by some practitioners because in the social world there are hectic variables that are impossible to control. Contextual problems require solutions geared to the precise situation rather than solutions that are general and context free. I would suggest there are few more hectic areas of practice than those encountered by nurses and so aptly described by Cox & Moss (1988) in their paper entitled 'The Chaos of Practice'. Schön's ability to appreciate this working world is a reason why his exposition on professional learning is so welcome to nurses.

Precise theories of safe drug administration are an example of espoused theories taught in class. In practice, however, a nurse may well decide, in the patient's best interest, to deviate in some way from the protocol. Some might counter that this example simply demonstrates that espoused theories in the real world should be used discriminately, as indeed Benner (1984) found expert nurses do. I would argue that it is this practical ability nurses have to use various sources of knowledge in a flexible way which is so impressive. This ability to discriminate 'on the job' is a clue to proficient and productive nursing, so eminently worth studying and encouraging through reflection on and in action.

Critical inquiry

Philosophically critical inquiry predominantly stems from the work of Habermas and other members of the Frankfurt School, although Carr & Kemmis (1986, p. 32) refer as far back as Aristotle when making their epistemological introduction to critical inquiry. Accordingly Carr & Kemmis (1986, pp. 33–34) support Aristotle's notion that the appropriateness of knowledge acquisition depends on the purpose that it serves. Habermas (1977) in similar vein describes three areas of human interest from which knowledge may arise.

These areas are *technical* interests that result in instrumental work guided by empirical knowledge; *practical* interests which are concerned with communication and intersubjectivity, guided by knowledge that provides understanding and lastly *emancipatory* interests which are concerned with social equity, freedom and justice guided by knowledge discovered through a process of conscientization. Freire (1972) explains conscientization as a dawning awareness, of competing human interests and power structures that, in effect, manufacture and perpetuate social situations. Mezirow (1981, p. 5) explains that the latter domain is termed emancipatory because it leads people to a true understanding of the cause of their predicaments and hopefully a pathway to their resolution of them.

Relating this last domain to nursing, as Carr & Kemmis (1986, p. 32) do to teaching, nurses develop competence through a process of critical reflection on experience, they examine their work and the contribution their nursing, and nursing generally, makes socially. Then in turn they also consider the effect social forces have upon themselves and their work. The notion of informed action or praxis is an important concept to critical theorists, one that is developed through the reciprocal relationship between action and critical reflection. The resulting heightened awareness and the revelation of the variety of factors that contribute to an established order can be used deliberately by people to understand, and in some instances rearrange, the social order in which they find themselves, in the name of justice and freedom.

By emancipation critical theorists refer to the freedom gained by people to contribute in a legitimate way to social systems that are equitable and just. The power to contribute equitably is achieved by those who learn how a situation is established and perpetuated. Emancipatory knowledge is gained from a broad perspective whereby issues are considered that are beyond the immediate situation such as the historical and political elements of the situation. Critical reflection involves Shor's (1987, p. 93) notion of the student *extraordinarily re-experiencing the ordinary*. This fresh view of everyday experience renders problematic things such as previously accepted value and belief systems and routines, generating questions such as, how are these ordinary things connected to economic, political and social exigencies? This new thinking can reveal distortions, that is those contributions, from unexpected sources, to the maintenance of the status quo. For instance students may come to appreciate their own contribution to a situation in which they are oppressed. Freire (1972, p. 376) suggests this type of knowledge (conscientization) equips people with the information needed to change situations radically, rather than to make superficial cosmetic alterations which serve in the long term to perpetuate injustice and allow current power relationships to persist.

Freire (1972) wrote of social revolution that would free both oppressors and the oppressed, but he warned against the possibility of the oppressed mimicking the behaviour of the oppressors, once the former obtained power. For it would then be likely that one oppressive system would replace another, and no lasting improvement be achieved. Whilst the critical theorists talk of social change, not all believe revolution is inevitable. Critical reflection will attune the student to the motives and perspectives of other parties in the social milieu, and this improved understanding of the situation may demonstrate that other interests, besides one's own, have a legitimate place in a just society.

Other theorists aligned to the critical approach are Marx and Freud. They are defined as critical because of Marx's notions of the critique of ideology (influential connected ideas that legitimize oppression), and because of Freud's psychoanalysis, whereby through self reflection the person can rediscover his or her self and the conditions they are in which may be repressive (Carr & Kemmis, 1986, p. 138). These sociological and psychological theories are good examples of how critical inquiry may lead to both personal growth and social improvement.

It is apparent that Schön's widely used work differs from the critical theorists. Schön concentrates predominantly on the development of the individual student's ability to address problems and develop skills in their particular context. He does not challenge the curriculum or call for social change. Adler (1991) notes for instance that Schön is predominantly interested in achieving the goals prescribed by the curriculum, for example learning to do the job efficiently. On the other hand whilst the critical theorists incorporate a responsibility for the broader social scene in their work, they are criticised for their impracticality. Besides raising consciousness they do not demonstrate how students might bring about change (Bell & Schniedewind, 1987).

An approach that incorporates the theories of Schön and the critical inquirers may be possible and may help to re-establish a balanced approach to nursing education in the following two areas. In the wake of the pervasive influence of humanistic ideas in recent times, nursing could be criticised for concentrating too much on the individual, rather than the collective problems of society. Bevis & Watson (1989) talk of the need for nurse education to find a balance between the focus on the individual micro perspective and the social macro perspective. Another balance needed is that between academic freedom, for example the freedom to pursue intellectual pathways that the individual deems appropriate, and the need for nursing students to acquire skills in order to protect the public from incompetent practitioners. These are problems we have to face and try to accommodate.

I am not suggesting that Schön's ideas and the work of critical theorists should be merged, there are too many differences for that. They may be used in a complementary fashion. Schön's techniques for learning practical skills and coaching students enables them to achieve competence in certain prescribed areas necessary to guarantee certain standards of professional work. The critical aspect incorporates a healthily sceptical view, (so necessary for critical thinking) of phenomena encountered in the educational process and encourages intellectual consideration of other options. It is a broader perspective that incorporates the students' search for an understanding of the social world and the ways in which this broader context affects them. It is only fair to help students to understand the differences between these two approaches to learning, in order that they can understand their role and objectives in the educational process using reflection for learning.

The pre-registration nursing courses are bound by the regulations of the statutory bodies to achieve certain standards and competencies, which means that some compromises have to be made in terms of the student's freedom to choose experience that is most meaningful to them. I would propose that curricula for advanced nursing courses need not be constrained by the need to acquire prescribed skills and that an emancipatory approach to learning could be adopted without compromise. Perhaps in some of the post-registration courses and course work for Master of Nursing degrees this should be considered. Wheeler & Chinn (1991) describe a feminist and emancipatory style of learning in which the group shares responsibility for devising the learning experience.

The process

The process of reflection for learning is dealt with in the educational literature, particularly explicitly in Schön (1987), Boud, Keogh & Walker (1985) and Boud & Walker (1991). Schön provides examples of students and coaches working together to analyse and learn from experience. Boud, Keogh & Walker (1985) have developed and refined (Boud & Walker, 1991) a model for reflective learning, which incorporates phases of preparation, experience, reflective processes and outcomes. Examples of recent nursing literature which, on the whole, has used the above authors' work and applied it to nursing situations are Emden (1991), Gray & Forsstrom (1991) and Cox, Hickson & Taylor (1991). Atkins and Murphy (1993, p. 1190) reviewed the literature on reflection and identify the skills most likely to be required for the process of reflection for learning. These skills range from self awareness to the following abilities: describe experiences; critically analyse situations; develop new perspectives and evaluate the learning process.

This type of learning is so personal it is doubtful that the literature can offer more than helpful suggestions. Readers will find that the other chapters in this book offer a great deal in terms of descriptions of how reflection for learning is carried out, as these accounts provide refreshing examples of unconventional and imaginative innovations. The literature however brings some issues to mind which are worth considering during the process of learning by reflection on experience.

The educationalists write of the potential difficulties that students will have reflecting critically and of the importance of expert support. Nursing students' difficulties are compounded in that they have to contend not only with dawning self awareness but practice situations in which they encounter a plethora of different emotions ranging from ecstatic relief to despair, fear, suffering, disgust and distress. It is good that nurses are encouraged to surface and examine their reactions to these phenomena through reflection. All too often in the past reactions have been repressed and must have contributed significantly to stress amongst nurses (Lawler, 1991; Smith, 1992). However these reactions can be expected and lecturers, mentors and lecturer-practitioners need to be prepared to support the students.

Much of Schön's work is carried out in safe situations. He describes the clinical practicum where situations are simulated and then reflected upon (Schön, 1987). This idea has not been adopted in Oxford, although in Australia the clinical laboratory has been retained. At Deakin University realistic scenarios of practice situations are performed in studios, or arts laboratories, by actors who are nursed by the students (Campbell, 1992). Following the scenario the students and actors discuss analytically all facets of the incident. This is an extension of the work Pearson undertook with the North West Spanner Group when working on the Nursing Development Unit in Burford (Pearson, Whitehouse & Morris, 1985). Allowing students to practise in the real situation at such an early stage (second year in Oxford) again emphasizes the need for adequate supervision.

Learning through reflection is a laborious and deliberate process. It does not just occur, nor is it something that is done in one's head on the way home. Thoughts on actions need to be articulated, either verbally or in writing. The work needs to be analysed critically, interpreted and compared with other perspectives. Schön (1987) describes reflective conversations where ideas are shared and debated, Boud, Keogh & Walker (1985) debriefing after experience and Holly (1987) keeping a professional journal. Space for this type of work needs to be built into the learning syllabus. It is hoped that there will come a time when reflection on action will be valued to such an extent that it can be given official time during the working day, when nurses can write about or discuss their experiences with the mutual purpose of learning from them.

Garrison (1991) writes that learning through reflection is a learning technique most suited to adults who have a wealth of past experience and an intellectual maturity to cope with autonomy, differing perspectives and shifting ideas. Even so, in Usher's (1985) experience most students initially find learning from experience strange. They are, on the whole, more comfortable learning facts from books.

There are a variety of reasons for these students' restricted view of learning, including issues such as past learning methods and traditional attitudes towards learning and education. Usher (1985) examines the issue of authority and suggests that however democratic a teacher wants to be they do exercise considerable authority and power in the learning situation. The sources of this power are the direction and outcome of the learning and the assessment of the student's progress. When the student does not have autonomy then it is likely that they will look to the teacher for direction and learn what they think the teacher wants them to rather than what seems most relevant to them.

This point is particularly relevant to nursing where students are given direction because certain competence is required in order to register and particularly so in Oxford where clinical practice is assessed and graded according to the student's ability to reflect critically upon their experience (Murphy & Reading, 1992, and see Chapter 2). Indeed in the second and third years students in Oxford seemed insecure and often asked for direction from mentors, personal tutors and lecturer-practitioners. Some direction is given to them in the form of specific competencies they need to master during the course; these competencies are not graded, they are either achieved at a minimum standard or not. A measure of freedom comes when the students are encouraged to reflect critically on their experiences and developing expertise and produce exemplars on their contracts. When writing their contracts they choose what examples to use themselves, there are no directives. However it is naive to think that the system is perfect and the degree of control over what nursing students learn is a potential obstruction to radical learning and out of tune with emancipatory pedagogy.

Nursing and reflection on experience

There is no doubt that reflection on action is an approach to learning that is gaining increasing popularity in the world of nursing. The appeal of reflective learning to the nursing profession has a number of sources, which involve areas such as nursing's history, ideologies and social circumstances.

In order to build a discipline and inform the profession, nurses are trying to find suitable means of knowledge acquisition, ways by which they can acknowledge and accommodate the subjective, unpredictable nature of the world in which they work. For a long time now, nurses have written of a growing sense of the limitations of traditional positivistic science. Schumacher and Gortner (1992) describe contemporary or post-positivistic thinking in the philosophy of science and suggest that arguments against the traditional science are somewhat late. Ideas in the philosophy of science are in a state of change and logical positivism is generally considered obsolete (Holmes (1991), Menke (1990), Schumacher & Gortner (1992)). Indeed there has been a trend since the 1960s to dismiss the notions of theory neutral observations, absolute truth and a static world as realistically impossible. This scepticism was encouraged by the work of the historicists notably Kuhn (1970) and Laudan (1977). Whilst I appreciate this point and believe that nurses have, as Holmes (1991) writes, been somewhat tardy in assimilating topical philosophical ideas, there is still evidence that traditional views remain dominant in practical spheres. This is especially so in the areas that impinge on the practical world of nurses, for example the style of research accepted by funding bodies and ethics committees, the style of management within the health service (which is still bureaucratic, medically dominated and product driven) and, relevant to this chapter, education. If nurses are to take new paths towards knowledge acquisition it is important for them to be able to explain and justify the practice discipline of nursing. This will be possible, it is suggested, if we investigate and thoroughly understand nursing practice.

Historically nurse education has been dominated by medical tradition and hence positivistic reductionist approaches. Evidence of this influence can be seen in old curricula with theory taught (often from other disciplines) and applied to practice. This perspective has contributed to the division of theory and practice (Munhall, 1982 and Alexander, 1983). Theories generated away from practice have been, on the whole unsuccessfully, applied to the practice situation. As Pearson (1992) also suggests, this traditional approach has led to the devaluation of the practice of nursing, as status is given to thinkers rather than doers. These problems have been recognized and deliberated upon by nurses for a long time, and as explained by Miller (1985), the means of over-coming them sought in a variety of ways. Cox *et al.* (1991, p. 374) proffer the notion that professional work and disciplinary knowledge are synergistic when, through praxis (thoughtful action), they actively complement one another.

In a concise exposition Schön (1983 and 1987) describes *the crisis in confidence in professional knowledge* (Schön, 1983, p. 3). There is a growing mistrust brought about by a suspicion that espoused theories from academia are inadequate for the preparation or continuing devel-opment of professional practitioners. There have been, and indeed still are, similar signs of dissatisfaction with nurse education manifest through the following groups: new practitioners who believe that their preparation was inadequate (UKCC, 1986); the anti-intellectual lobby, 'you don't need degrees to nurse, what's wrong with good old-fashioned caring'; the frustrated nursing students reading for post-registration certificates and degrees who find their study material divorced from their reality and lastly the relatively slow development and appreciation of the discipline of nursing by nurses at all levels in practice institutions.

Whilst it can be argued that all these parties have some flaws in their arguments, and are at times critical in an irresponsible way, it is reasonable that nurses should wish academics and educationalists to pay attention to their actions. Most nurses wish to have their consider-able abilities appreciated and used to contribute to the growing body of knowledge for the discipline of nursing. However this will only be achieved when it is possible to make explicit what it is nurses do so well. Benner (1984) and Benner & Wrubel (1989) have done a great deal through their phenomenological research to clarify and enhance the value of the art of expert nursing. This type of clarity can be obtained, suggest Perry & Moss (1989), by practitioners who are prepared to examine their work in a critically reflective way. Reflection on action in writing, conversations and discussions should help nurses to develop the ability to articulate their craft.

Lumby (1991 and 1992) eloquently explains the need for nurses to develop a language of nursing to express the discipline adequately – a language that accommodates an appreciation of the subjective, wonderful and unpredictable nature of the world and which provides a means to justify fair and meaningful ways of sharing and evaluating nursing work. Familiar 'scientific' language has limited nurses by words, like 'sample', 'objectivity', 'generalizability' and 'validity'. These words are classically used to justify experimental work and do not suit the interpretive and creative work nurses are generating. What is required is syntax that portrays the exquisite sensitivity of the art and science of nursing and that denotes its unique world. Lumby (1991) exhorts nurses to identify and publicly discuss nursing praxis, exercising, refining and developing our rhetoric, otherwise we may remain constrained in the world of medicine. Reflection on and in action is an essential fuel for such conversations.

Popular and persuasive ideas amongst nurses are that the practice of nursing is the focus of the discipline (Benner (1984), Watson (1985), Pearson (1988, 1991 and 1992), Gray & Forsstrom (1991)) and an important source of knowledge. Cox *et al.* (1991, p. 373) describe nursing as 'careful people-orientated work, which is energised by knowledge', a knowledge that is embedded in the practice of nursing. Attention turned upon nursing work, one example of which is critical reflection on action, is most appropriate for the generation and acquisition of contemporary nursing knowledge.

New courses in the tertiary education sector have resulted in standards which require that nurses are adequately prepared to practise and furthermore to pursue practice in an intellectual way (Oxford Polytechnic, 1988). Critical reflection upon practice appears to be an appropriate approach to combine an appreciation for action and critical inquiry in an academically and practically acceptable way.

Emden (1991) contends that a responsible aspiration of all mature nurses is to become a reflective practitioner capable of improving practice by asking difficult questions and being sceptical of practices taken for granted. She describes a process of empowerment and emancipation through critical awareness of an individual's nursing work and situation. Furthermore it is a process which is also useful for members of nursing faculties who continue to develop their practice knowledge as well as their nursing expertise.

Gray & Forsstrom (1991, p. 355) describe a project where they used 'the reflective technique' to generate theory from practice on regular faculty practice days. The issue of faculty practice is another one which has perplexed the profession for quite a time. It is problematic that so much nursing is taught by people who no longer practise, for they are deprived of an important source of nursing knowledge. Their critical reflections on nursing practice are sometimes of a second hand nature making it difficult for lecturers to gain credibility. Yet the practical problems of faculty practice are complex and mere presence in the workplace is certainly not enough to advance lecturers' knowledge of nursing. Gray & Forsstrom's work (1991) is a useful introduction to reflective practice for lecturers and has great potential for making faculty practice meaningful, besides enabling lecturers to understand the nature of reflective nursing practice which they are encouraging in nursing students. The pertinence of this work will be apparent as lecturers start to nurse therapeutically and are able to reflect critically on their own expertise. They will became therapists when they devise more flexible times and creative methods of practice, offering clients expertise and continuity of service.

On a political tack nurses are reviewing their predicament which can appear 'irrational, unjust and unfulfilling' (Emden, 1991, p. 348). One example is the exploration of the effects medical dominance has, and has had on the development of the mainly female profession of nursing (Salvage (1985), Lumby (1991), Short, Sharman & Speedy (1992)). A critical social view of nursing reveals, through reflection, distortions and inequalities in the system, exposes power relationships and clarifies routes for collaborative change. Nurses are quite aware that in the current political climate they desperately need to understand the complex local, national and international situations of nurses in order to secure a proper contribution in the changing health care system. It is understood that this process of emancipation may well demonstrate the contributions nurses make to their own oppression in the system.

Whilst these reasons for adopting reflection on experience for nursing study are persuasive some cautions are wisely raised in both nursing and educational literature. These cautions are of a practical, political, philosophical and moral nature.

It can appear that reflection is easy and something which the students can be sent off to do. However reflection is a process of gradual self awareness, critical appraisal of the social world and transformation. These are not particularly comfortable processes, which may lead students to personal distress and conflict. Reflective practitioners need handy encouragement and professional help. In Oxford, students work with mentors, who are themselves reflective practitioners and have been educationally prepared for the role of helping nursing undergraduates. The students and mentors are guided and supported by lecturer-practitioners, ideally and usually in the student's immediate clinical area. This system is laborious and it is most likely that any other scheme to provide adequate support and supervision to students learning through reflection on practice will have similar resource implications.

There is perhaps a modern tendency to romanticize nursing practice. It is comfortable to imagine that all nurses are the ingenious carers as described by Benner (1984), however it should be remembered that she investigated 'expert practice'. There would be doubtful benefits if reflection on action gave some nurses the excuse to validate their current practice and ignore theory or continuing education altogether. There are nurses who have cruised through their careers picking up knowledge in an effortless and haphazard way and they may incorrectly relate this process to reflection. Whilst some of the knowledge they gain will be practical, their lack of self criticism means that in their work they probably propound some myths, unchallenged attitudes and outdated practices too. The process of reflection is hard work and involves a commitment of both time and intellectual effort in order for the practitioner to progress. It is not something done unintentionally or effortlessly.

Griffiths & Tann (1992) raise the issue of political pressure on professions. The notion of learning on the job for teacher education has appealed to politicians and given some of them an excuse to criticize the colleges of education. Ideas are emerging that all students need is a mentor in practice to show them the ropes, therefore the faculty and investment in the colleges can be reduced. Politicians have berated educationalists for being too theoretical and the source of outlandish and unsuccessful experiments in education. It is possible that similar pressure could be put on nurses to return to basics and turn from academia to the bed side. Moves to increase experiential learning methods to disproportionate levels within theoretical courses are probably premature as the results of learning from experience as reflective practitioners in education are mainly disappointing to date (Griffiths & Tann, 1992). Besides, learning through reflection on experience is not purely experiential as Griffiths & Tann (1992) point out – students are still required to study relevant theories and search the literature in order to augment their own thoughts.

The use of emancipatory critical theory raises some moral issues. It is not apparent that students and quite often lecturers are aware that critical reflection will almost inevitably lead the student to challenge and change the status quo. Even in the early days Oxford nursing students were creating dissonance in both the practice and educational institutions. Some would applaud this as it is about time nurses questioned practice and brought about changes in some traditional spheres. However, it is appropriate to question how fair it is that neophytes are set up to do this difficult work without adequate preparation or indeed authority. Freire (1972) warns of the disillusion experienced by the oppressed who identify the sources of their oppression and yet are still powerless to make a difference.

Emancipation through critical reflection requires a considerable degree of maturity, for the student is required to reframe personal perspectives – to see situations in new ways, not necessarily always from their perspective. Other parties' points of view need to be considered as fairly as possible in order to build up a comprehensive social picture. It is likely that nurses contribute to their own oppression and the oppression of others. Perspective transformation (change in personal perspective) is required to deal with others in a fair and equitable manner. Premature mounting of personal or professional soap boxes is not a reasonable goal for the critically reflective practitioner, but one I fear that may be all too easy to achieve if care is not taken to avoid this narrow perspective.

So reflection on experience and critical reflection may enable nurses to focus on practice and give it the premier status within the discipline. They may find it a useful pathway to the generation and articulation of knowledge specific and practically useful to nursing in both clinical and academic institutions. It may also provide the means for nurses to understand and contribute towards change in their social world. These are optimistic assertions indeed which should be tempered with cautions. Reflection is not a panacea for nursing's many dilemmas – it is a way of learning more about our work. Whatever method is chosen for learning the important factors will always be the individual's ability and commitment to learn and the conduciveness of the learning institution.

Research

To date I do not know of any nursing research studies, aside from Powell's (1991) study, that relate directly to reflection and the education of nurses. There are however, a few studies which have taken a critical approach in investigating the practice worlds of nursing (Perry (1985), Hickson (1988) and Street (1992)). On the whole I think that this paucity is probably reasonable in view of the relatively recent introduction of reflection for learning to nursing curricula. The hiatus may give nurses a chance to really think about the most appropriate ways to explore reflection as a learning method for nurses.

I hope that nursing researchers investigating reflection will not be enticed down the traditional path of measurement, comparison and evaluation. If they do they will come across the same problems that researchers have had with nursing models (Silva, 1977) and primary nursing (Giovanetti, 1986). They found that it was impossible to control variables in the complex and ever changing nursing world. The values and beliefs regarding knowledge acquisition that underpin positivistic research methods are contradictory to those of the subject of their research. It is not possible to do justice to critical reflection when applying traditional scientific criteria and language to students' progress and outcomes when its philosophical foundations, as I hope I have demonstrated in this chapter, are quite different.

We hope this book may be a useful, if an unconventional, starting point for intellectual thought regarding reflection as a learning method for nursing. In these chapters expositions of our early experiences are written which are an important first step towards an understanding of the impact the use of critical reflection has in nurse education. Nurses from the School of Health Care Studies at Oxford Brookes University intend to continue research projects that explore critical reflection, a learning method that has been a standard part of our courses and practice since the inception of the school.

I suspect that the process of reflective learning, rather than the product, may be the most informative field for research. Usher (1985) and Garrison (1991) stress that the process of learning from reflection on experience is as important as the product. Anecdotes provide clues to interesting paths researchers may wish to pursue. For instance, a lecturer from another university reported that 'Deakin nurses were obviously used to reflection on action and could always be relied upon to tell a good story'. What were these stories? What did they say about practice? What effect did they have in practice? A third year Oxford nursing student once explained to me how more mature the nursing students had become compared to students from other courses in the University. She related this maturity to the personal development she had acquired through critical reflection of her practice. What was this maturity? How did it develop? How did she demonstrate it both socially and professionally? I am sure that the chapters in the book will throw open many other questions worth examining through research.

What may be confusing to some is that critical reflection is an integral part of emancipatory or critical inquiry methodologies. Smith (1990, p. 177) lists these methodologies within the critical paradigm as 'critical praxis, research-as-praxis, emancipatory research, action research, and critical ethnography'. These approaches all have components where critical theorems arise from the research participants' critical reflection of the information collected. This process reveals power relationships, particular interests and distortions that compound the particular practical situation under scrutiny. It is argued, albeit in a less deliberate way, that nurses who use critical reflection on their actions, as a method of understanding their work, are akin to researchers generating theories.

Usher (1985), Cox *et al.* (1991) and Griffiths & Tann (1992) discuss the relationship between personal knowledge generated from individual experience and theories that are derived from literature. Usher (1985, p. 103) explains that they simply represent different perspectives and together knowledge derived in these different ways complement the total view of the problem under scrutiny. Cox *et al.* (1991, p. 388) agree but proceed further in explaining how theories generated professionally from experience and enacted in the nursing situation are an important contribution to the disciplinary knowledge of nursing. Important because they represent the essential nature of nursing practice.

Conclusion

Boud & Walker (1991) believe that people need to be able to learn from their experience in order to accept positions of responsibility. The process of learning to learn from experience is as important as the end product of the learning, namely an ability to view a phenomenon from a different perspective and translate new knowledge into action. The process is important because it equips the professional to meet various practical problems and deal with them intelligently – a necessary requirement for all nurses. This is especially so as nursing changes to meet the demands of society as the year 2000 approaches. No longer are nurses training to work just in hospitals – they will work in many different areas and it is to be hoped that their critical ability will enable them to appraise new work and identify what needs to be learnt, challenged, altered and further investigated in any nursing context.

As is usual with fashions in nursing there are many expectations and high hopes for benefits to be gained by this style of learning. Some of these benefits have been considered in this chapter. However it would be an optimist indeed who really believed that critical reflection alone could bring about such radical improvements. Reflection on experience is a path worth pursuing for it leads in the right direction: towards an education where nurses learn to understand the meaning of their experiences, towards a profession that values its practical expertise, towards a research tradition that has a language that adequately expresses nursing work and finally towards a discipline whose knowledge is not only embedded in nursing practice but can be expressed in new and transforming ways.

References

Adler, S. (1991 The reflective practitioner and the curriculum of teacher education. *Journal of Education for Teaching,* **17**, No. 2, 139–50.

Alexander, M.F. (1983) *Learning to Nurse,* Churchill Livingstone, Edinburgh.

Argyris, C. & Schön, D. (1974) *Theory in Practice: Increasing Professional Effectiveness,* Jossey-Bass, San Francisco.

Argyris, C. & Schön, D. (1978) *Organisational Learning.* Addison-Wesley, Massachusetts.

Atkins, S. & Murphy, C. (1993) Reflection: a review of the literature. *Journal of Advanced Nursing,* **18**, No. 8, 1188–92.

Bell, L. & Schniedewind, N. (1987) Reflective minds/intentional hearts: joining humanistic education and critical theory for liberating education *Journal of Education,* **169**, 2, 55–78.

Benner, P. (1984) *From Novice to Expert: Excellence and Power in Clinical Nursing Practice,* Addison-Wesley, California.

Benner, P. & Wrubel, J. (1989) *The Primacy of Caring: Stress and Coping in Health and Illness,* Addison-Wesley, California.

Bevis, E. & Watson, J. (1989) *Toward a Caring Curriculum: A New Pedagogy for Nursing,* National League for Nursing, New York.

Boud, D., Keogh, R. & Walker, D. (1985) *Reflection: Turning Experience into Learning,* Kogan Page, London.

Boud, D. & Walker, D. (1991) *Experiencing and Learning: Reflection at Work,* Deakin University Press, Geelong.

Campbell, I. (1992) Myriad – The use of arts as a reflective process in nurse education. Paper presented at the Royal College of Australia First National Nursing Forum *Nursing Kaleidoscope: Sharpen the Focus,* Adelaide.

Carr, W. & Kemmis, S. (1986) *Becoming Critical: Education, Knowledge and Action Research,* The Falmer Press, London.

Champion, R. (1992) The philosophy of an honours degree program in nursing and midwifery. In Bines, H. & Watson, D. (Eds.) *Developing Professional Education.* Society for Research into Higher Education & Open University Press, Milton Keynes.

Clarke, M. (1986) Action and reflection: practice and theory in nursing. *Journal of Advanced Nursing,* **11**, 3–11.

Cox, H. & Moss, C. (1988) Promiscuous knowledge: the chaos of practice. The Olive Anstey Nursing Foundation International Conference: Promiscuous Knowledge. Perth.

Cox, H., Hickson, P. & Taylor, B. (1991) Exploring reflection: Knowing and constructing practice. In Grey, G. & Pratt, R. *Towards a Discipline of Nursing,* Churchill Livingstone, Melbourne.

Deakin University (1988) *Diploma of Nursing: Curriculum Document,* Deakin School of Nursing, Geelong.

Descartes, R. (1984) The Search for Truth. In *The Philosophical Writings of Descartes,* Vol 2, Cottingham, J., Stoothoff, R. & Murdoch, D. (trs.) Cambridge University Press, Cambridge.

Dewey, J. (1933) *How We Think,* D.C. Heath, Boston.

Emden, C. (1991) Becoming a reflective practitioner. In Gray, G. & Pratt, R. *Towards a Discipline of Nursing,* Churchill Livingstone, Melbourne.

Freire, P. (1972) *Pedagogy of the Oppressed.* Penguin Books, Harmondsworth.

Garrison, D. (1991) Critical thinking and adult education: a conceptual model for developing critical thinking in adult learners. *International Journal of Lifelong Education,* **10**, No 4, 287–303.

George, P. (1986) The Nurse as a Reflective Practitioner. Unpublished paper, Oxford Polytechnic, Oxford.

Giovanetti, P. (1986) Evaluation of Primary Nursing. In Weilty, H., Fitzpatrick, J. & Taundon, J. *The Annual Review of Nursing Research*, Springer Publishing Company, New York.

Gray, J. & Forsstrom, S. (1991) Generating theory from practice: the reflective technique. Chapter in Gray, G. & Pratt, R. *Towards a Discipline of Nursing*, Churchill Livingstone, Melbourne.

Griffiths, M. & Tann, S. (1992) Using reflective practice to link personal and public theories. *Journal of Education for Teaching*, **18**, No. 1, 69–84.

Habermas, J. (1977) *Knowledge and Human Interests*, Beacon Press, Boston.

Hickson, P. (1988) *Knowledge and action in nursing: a critical approach to the practice worlds of four nurses.* Unpublished Masters Thesis, Massey University, Toronto.

Holly, M. (1987) *Keeping a personal-professional journal.* Revised Edition, Deakin University Press, Geelong.

Holmes, C. (1991) Theory: Where are we going and what have we missed along the way? In Gray, G. and Pratt, R. *Towards a Discipline of Nursing*, Churchill Livingstone, Melbourne.

Kuhn, T. (1970) *The Structure of Scientific Revolutions*, 2nd edition, University of Chicago Press, Chicago.

Laudan, L. (1977) *Progress and Its Problems: Towards a Theory of Scientific Growth*, University of California, Berkeley.

Lawler, J. (1991) *Behind the Screens Nursing Comology, the Problem of the Body*, Churchill Livingstone, Melbourne.

Lumby, J. (1991) Threads of an emerging discipline. In Gray, G. & Pratt, R. *Towards a Discipline of Nursing*, Churchill Livingstone, Melbourne.

Lumby, J. (1992) Re-emergence of Vision. Paper presented at The Royal College of Nursing Australia First National Nursing Forum, *Nursing Kaleidoscope: Sharpen the Focus*, Adelaide, June.

Macquarie Dictionary (1991) *The Macquarie Dictionary.* 2nd edition. Macquarie Library Pty Ltd, Sydney.

Menke, E. (1983) Critical analysis of theory development in nursing. In Chaska, N. (ed.) *The Nursing Profession*, McGraw Hill, New York.

Mezirow, J. (1981) A critical theory of adult learning and education, *Adult Education* 32 No. 1, 3–24.

Miller, A. (1985) The relationship between nursing theory and nursing practice. *Journal of Advanced Nursing*, **10**, 414–24.

Munhall, P.L. (1982) Nursing philosophy and nursing research: in apposition or opposition? *Nursing Research*, **31**, No. 3, 176–7, 181.

Murphy, C. & Reading, P. (1992) Assessing professional competence. In Bines, H. & Watson, D. (Eds.) *Developing Professional Education.* Society for Research into Higher Education & Open University Press, Buckingham.

Newell, R. (1992) Anxiety, accuracy and reflection: the limits of professional development *Journal of Advanced Nursing*, **17**, 1326–33.

Oxford Polytechnic, Department of Nursing, Midwifery and Health Visiting (1988) Submission of course proposals. Unpublished.

Pearson, A., Whitehouse, C. & Morris, P. (1985) Consumer orientated groups: a new approach to interdisciplinary teaching. *Journal of the Royal College of Practitioners*, **35**, 381–3.

Pearson, A. (1988) *Primary Nursing – Nursing in the Burford and Oxford Nursing Development Units*, Croom Helm, London.

Pearson, A. (1991). Nursing as Caring. In McMahon, R. & Pearson, A. *Nursing as Therapy*. Chapman & Hall, London.

Pearson, A. (1992) Knowing nursing: emerging paradigms in nursing. In Robinson, K. & Vaughan, B. (Eds.) *Knowledge for Nursing Practice*. John Wiley, London.

Perry, J. (1985) *Theory & practice in the induction of five graduate nurses: a reflexive critique*, Masters Thesis, Massey University, Toronto.

Perry, J. & Moss, C. (1989) Generating alternatives in nursing: turning curriculum into a living process. *The Australian Journal of Advanced Nursing*, **6**, 2, 35–40.

Powell, J. (1991) Reflection and the evaluation of experience: prerequisites for therapeutic practice. In McMahon, R. & Pearson, A. *Nursing as Therapy*. Chapman & Hall, London.

Robinson, K. & Vaughan, B. (1992) *Knowledge for Nursing Practice*. John Wiley, London.

Salvage, J. (1985) *The Politics of Nursing*. Heinemann, London.

Sater, B. (1988) *The Stream of Becoming: A Study of Martha Roger's Theory*. National League for Nursing, New York.

Schön, D. (1983) *The Reflective Practitioner*. Basic Books Harper Collins, San Francisco.

Schön, D. (1987) *Educating the Reflective Practitioner*. Jossey-Bass Publishers, San Francisco.

Schumacher, K. & Gortner, S. (1992) (Mis) conceptions and reconceptions about traditional science. *Advances in Nursing Science*, **14**(4), 1–11.

Shapiro, S. (1991) The end of radical hope? Postmodernism and the challenge to critical pedagogy. *Education and Society*, **9** No. 2, 112–22.

Shor, I. (1987) *Critical Teaching and Everyday Life*, University of Chicago Press, Chicago.

Short, S., Sharman, E. & Speedy,S. (1992) *Sociology for Nurses*, Macmillan, London.

Silva, M. (1977) Philosophy, science, theory: interrelationships and implications for nursing research. *Image* **9**, 59–63.

Smith, B. (1990) The critical approach. In Smith, B., Connole, H., Speedy, S. and Wisean, R. *Issues and Methods in Research Study Guide*, South Australian College of Advanced Education, Adelaide.

Smith, P. (1992) *The Emotional Labour of Nursing: How Nurses Care*, Macmillan, London.

Smyth, W. (1986) *Reflection in Action*. Deakin University Press, Geelong.

Street, A. (1988) *Nursing Practice: High, hard ground, messy swamps and the pathways in between*. Deakin University Press, Geelong.

Street, A. (1992) *Inside Nursing: a Critical Ethnography of Clinical Nursing Practice*. Suny Cornhill.

Turner, B. (1990) *Theories of Modernity and Post Modernity*, Sage Publications, San Mateo.

UKCC (1986) *Project 2000: A New Preparation for Practice*, United Kingdom Central Council for Nursing, Midwifery and Health Visiting, London.

Usher, R. (1985) Beyond the anecdotal: adult learning and the use of experience. *Studies in the Education of Adults*, **17** No 1, pp 59–74.

Watson, J. (1985) *Nursing – the Philosophy and Science of Caring*. Colorado Associated University Press, Denver.

Wheeler, C. & Chinn, P. (1991) *Peace and Power: A Handbook of Feminist Process*, 3rd Edition. National League for Nurses, New York.

Chapter 6
Pushing Back the Boundaries of Personal Experience

Introduction

This chapter is a personal exploration of the value of reflection as an educational approach to developing my nursing practice. It is an approach that I have actively and consciously applied intermittently to all aspects of my nursing for many years now. The focus of this chapter is the clinical side of my nursing and as a strategy for learning I find reflection equally helpful in all other aspects of my life.

My understanding of nursing when I qualified was both naive and simplistic. I saw nursing as caring for people in distress. At this time that meant doing things for people in a skilful, sympathetic and efficient manner. My understanding of and beliefs about nursing have changed dramatically since then. The view that I now subscribe to is most clearly articulated by Paterson & Zderad (1976) who see nursing as the nurturing response of one person to another in need. McKee (1991) describes the aim of nursing 'to develop human potential to its utmost: its goal is well-being and more-being'. She describes nursing as 'a lived experienced, a response to a human situation which the nurse shares with another'.

I believe that it is far more than the passage of time which has matured my understanding of what nursing is and can be. I believe that my new perspective grew from my struggle to understand the meaning of the lived experience of nursing. The vehicle for this journey was the experience of reflection upon my nursing actions.

I hope that by answering the four questions most commonly asked of me with regard to reflection I will be able to share my experience of becoming a reflective practitioner of nursing.

- How does reflection enrich my practice?
- What qualities does a reflective practitioner require?
- What is needed to become a more skilful reflective practitioner?
- How do I reflect?

Having explored these questions I shall attempt to make the general issues raised much more specific by reflecting on an exemplar from my practice and illustrating what can be learnt about one's nursing practice by doing so.

How does reflection enrich my practice?

As I gain more experience as a practitioner I find that I am increasingly able to articulate my personal philosophy of nursing. I know the values, attitudes and beliefs that guide my practice. What is much harder to determine is whether these concepts are discernible from my daily actions. I find reflection invaluable in helping me to assess if my behaviour is congruent with my professed values and beliefs. I feel that without this self monitoring ability it would be impossible for me to know with certainty if the reality of my practice lived up to my aspirations. At times my reflections upon my actions do reveal a dissonance, for example patient autonomy is a concept that I try to make an integral part of my nursing practice but occasionally I find myself telling patients what I think they should do. I suppose old habits die hard and it is much easier to know what you should be doing than to do it. I think that I would find it extremely difficult to detect this contradiction within my nursing practice without reflection upon the meaning of my everyday actions. It is reassuring that reflection develops the ability to be specific about what new knowledge of myself or the situation I have uncovered and to explore the future implications of this for my practice.

One of the most powerful effects of regularly reflecting upon my clinical practice is that it prevents me from becoming complacent with everyday aspects of my work. Jarvis (1987) recognises the potential for any action that is repeatedly practised to become habitualized. He sees reflection on action as a valuable way of safeguarding practice from becoming mindless and ritualized.

Reflection is extremely effective in increasing my focus upon aspects of nursing care that could be taken for granted. By regularly analysing apparently insignificant details of clinical care I can maintain my focus upon the meaning of that event to the patient. Examples of such events could be a patient needing help with feeding, or helping someone onto the toilet. Reflection in action increases the level of consciousness required to perform any element of care and supports the unique nature of any interaction within the situation. It is this willingness to explore the meaning of the event from the patients' perspective that prevents these actions from becoming ritualised.

I have found that reflecting in action has increased my ability to look upon my world with eyes other than my own. It develops the ability to explore situations from another's perspective. To reflect upon an event it is important not only to include information of your understanding but also information from the viewpoint of every other participant in that event. I find that this skill is particularly valuable when one considers the role of the nurse in our present health care system. I work within many different teams, some of which are only very loosely defined. There is a difference in how well individuals know one another, for example there is consistent membership of the nursing team that I work within but an ever changing membership of the multidisciplinary team that may be required to plan a successful discharge. This is because different professionals will be involved dependent upon the patient's specific needs. I believe that it is important to know how others perceive my actions. Not just my patients, but colleagues from all professions.

Reflection has been a specific help in developing my understanding of complex interpersonal and interprofessional situations. There have been incidents which if I had not reflected upon them would have left me with unresolved feelings that would have influenced my future behaviour without me perhaps ever knowing why. By reflecting on these incidents I can untangle the different aspects of each event and learn why the incident evolved as it did. This is vitally important because it helps me to recognise what my role was in a situation and to pinpoint actions that were particularly skilful, or not. Without this insight and understanding of the meaning of the events and the part I have played in them I would not have the opportunity to learn from them. I believe this to be particularly important in relation to events that I am left with very strong negative feelings about. The understanding that comes through reflection helps to place even the most powerful experiences into perspective.

Through the process of reflection I have the ability to recognise aspects of my behaviour that are not helpful to developing the style of nursing that I aspire to. This self awareness, whilst not solving the problem, does enable me to develop a strategy for limiting its effect upon my practice. It also allows me to identify particular skills that I do have, thereby increasing the likelihood that I will be able to use them more consciously in the future.

The analytical skills that I have developed through reflection are particularly useful in helping me to recognize and value different types of knowledge that are necessary to nurse expertly. I now realize that before I began to reflect on my nursing practice the only type of knowledge that I recognized and understood was that which Carper (1978) describes as empirical and ethical. This I believe reflects my individual education up to that time which was based upon a model of technical rationality (Schön, 1983). I realize that even at this time I did not feel as if the knowledge I had equipped me for the work that I would be doing, or the decisions that I would be making. I rationalized this by telling myself that all would become clear when I had some more experience of nursing. As time passed and I gained experience it helped to some extent, but not as much as I had hoped.

Donald Schön's (1983) work on reflection in action helped me to understand my inner disharmony and to recognize artistic knowledge and self knowledge. These forms of knowledge are also described by Carper (1978) as aesthetic and personal knowledge. Until this time I had not appreciated the value of these forms of knowing in relation to my professional practice. Again, through the experience of reflection on and in action I recognized the potential for developing and understanding my nursing that this broader view of knowledge had given me.

Until this time I did not understand quite how strongly how who I was influenced how I nursed. I now believe that self knowledge and aesthetic knowledge are just as important as empirical and ethical knowledge if I am to deliver a high quality of care to my patients. I value all life experiences as having the power to influence my practice. Some of the most painful experiences in my personal life have resulted in the most significant developments in my nursing practice. Similarly upsetting negative experiences of practice, through reflection have generated uncomfortable but significant learning outcomes. These have been difficult but vital lessons in understanding the inner meaning of nursing. I do not believe that these personal events would necessarily have influenced my practice to such a degree without my ability to learn through structured reflection upon my experience.

Street (1990) speaks of the awesome complexity of clinical nursing, where every problem is unique. This is certainly true in relation to any problem that is interpreted from the patient's perspective. I have found traditional scientific theory woefully lacking in helping to solve such problems. Schön (1987) describes professional practice as having 'a varied topography consisting of high ground overlooking a swamp of clinical practice'. The high dry ground is the domain of technical rationality and is where simple technical problems lie. The murky swamps are the territory of the almost indefinable intricate problems of clinical practice. Schön advocates the use of reflection in action to help professionals to define and solve these unique problems.

A certain freedom is created with the realization that you have the skills to analyse an intricate problem, to untangle the web and get to the heart of the matter. I have found that most of the murkiness in the swamp that Schön speaks of comes from an inability to see clearly. This relates to the difficulty in identifying a patient's problem accurately. Reflection has given me the ability to see much more clearly whilst I am in the swamp. The increased awareness of my knowledge and skills allows me to tread a delicate path once I have recognized where I need to go. I believe that reflection has broadened my vision of what is possible, it has increased my confidence so that I no longer have to cut the situation to fit my professional knowledge (Schön, 1987). This allows me to practise in a manner that is focused on the meaning of the situation to my patient.

I have found that the process of reflection in action allows me to be creative in solving these unique clinical problems. I have learnt to recognize key elements of similar experiences and combine them into innovative solutions individually designed for each new problem. The confidence that comes from accepting that I do not have to find neat nursing solutions to every problem gives me the freedom to work with my patients identifying what they feel their problems are. In this way I allow my patients to show me the kind of care that they need to achieve a state of well being.

What qualities does a reflective practitioner require?

If I had to identify three personal attributes that were vital to becoming a reflecting practitioner these would be commitment, energy and a willingness to learn. I think that a commitment to develop your nursing practice is the most important prerequisite for becoming a reflective practitioner. This is because learning through reflection is a skill, and as such is not perfected instantly. The rewards of reflection really begin to emerge as this skill gets refined. When I first began to reflect upon my practice I invariably uncovered more questions than new meanings and insight. With commitment and perseverance I can now learn an astonishing amount about myself and others through the conscious use of reflection. Dewey (1933) expresses the above in terms of a responsibility to search for the meaning within a situation. I see this in relation to a search for the consequences and implications of my clinical actions. It helps to expand my vision of the potential effects of any action that I take.

Reflection is far more than a thoughtful approach to nursing, it is more a way of being, a state of mind. Reflection is not passive contemplation, it is an active process and as such requires energy to flourish. This is something that I was aware of but did not truly believe until I had experienced it for myself. I find it exhausting to explore an area of practice and come face to face with the unpredictability and uncertainty of it. It then takes courage to recognize that there are no neat solutions, and that you must use elements of past experiences selectively to generate new strategies.

I believe that a reflective practitioner requires the ability to balance idealism and realism. I see reflection as an extremely useful tool to help me strive to attain my ideals whilst helping me to understand why I have not reached them. This requires a certain pragmatism and maturity of character. Reflection does reveal aspects of your personality or behaviour in particular situations that you may not be proud of. I believe that one must have an internal maturity and external support to be able to undertake this kind of learning. The energy and maturity that I have described are expressed by Dewey (1933) as a wholeheartedness. I see this as an inner strength that allows me to subject myself to the scrutiny of reflection because I value the outcome.

The third part of this basic kit for reflection is a willingness to learn, about yourself and your practice. This is analogous to Dewey's (1933) concept of openmindedness. It is an attitude that I find helps me to try to see a situation from a perspective other than my own, to listen to another's viewpoint, regardless of who they are. It enables me to examine rationales that underlie areas of my practice that I may take for granted and not to feel threatened when others do the same. I have found that in the context of my working life this is much easier to talk about than to achieve in practice! I find that I often need a cooling off period to allow my feelings to settle before I can reflect upon a complex situation with any degree of openmindedness.

In the seven years that I have been developing the skill of reflection I feel that I have probably learnt more about myself than about nursing. However this self knowledge had transformed my practice more than I could have thought possible at the outset. This willingness to learn is apparent also in the questions that I am able to put to myself. There is no area of my nursing that is excluded from this reflective scrutiny. No belief or technique is too precious to be challenged. I am certain that what makes this possible is the fact that it is a challenge from within. It is difficult to remain defensive in response to a question that you have asked yourself, because you cannot fool yourself convincingly indefinitely. At times though I have found that you cannot force yourself to recognize certain truths until you are ready to. I believe that to do so would be wrong.

What is needed to become a more reflective practitioner?

So far I feel that I have focused very much upon reflection as an individual activity. This does not give the full picture. Just as nursing cannot happen in social isolation, nor should reflection. I have found that although I do learn about myself through individual reflection, my most valuable insights have been gained by including others in this process. I feel that in addition to exploring individual qualities and strengths, consideration should also be paid to the social context of any nursing action.

In response to the question of what is needed to become a more reflective practitioner, I would say very strongly, the company of others. I have found that the social and professional climate of the workplace are vitally important in relation to the way my practice develops. I have emphasised the benefits of self knowledge gained through reflection, and intimated that this is not always a comfortable experience. Sometimes it is downright painful and it is important to work with people who will support you through the difficult times and celebrate in the good.

In my mind a suitable environment to encourage reflection is one that is committed to professional practice; where every individual is consciously trying to develop their nursing practice, and the concept of teamwork is well established. My nursing practice has progressed most rapidly at times when I have had the company of like minded individuals who have similar beliefs and values regarding nursing. Working relationships that are based upon trust and mutual respect lead to the opportunity for innovative practice to thrive. It is when I have been part of such teams that I have received the appropriate level of support and challenge to reflect fully upon my nursing actions. Obviously the best possible environment would be one where colleagues are not only committed to professional practice but also to becoming reflective practitioners. To be part of such a team is exhilarating though demanding. In such a team colleagues understand the value of accurate feedback, encouragement, and support in clinical risk taking. They also recognize that time spent at work discussing nursing and shared experiences of nursing is not time wasted. They recognize the value of not just nursing action but reflection upon nursing action. In such an environment the emphasis of priorities change. Obviously all aspects of care must still be carried out but the emphasis is also upon 'what is the meaning of what has been done'.

How do I reflect?

Learning through reflection is an individual process. People can give advice and hints and tips, but you only really learn by having a go. A particular method or strategy that works for one person may be a hindrance to another. What follows therefore is a personal account of what works for me.

I am aware that I have a fairly eclectic approach to reflecting upon my nursing practice. This is not necessarily a bad thing, because different situations call for different approaches to understanding them. However, I do feel that you need to strike a balance between having access to a variety of methods of reflection and developing the ability to reflect skilfully and in depth using one particular approach.

My reflective journal is particularly important to me, it is now a precious record of the highs and lows of my nursing experience. These vivid episodes are separated by numerous almost incidental moments that I have recorded and reflected upon. I try to write in my journal twice a week, however some weeks I do not write at all. It is usually when life is particularly chaotic or depressing that I cannot discipline myself to find the time or energy to write. It is ironic that this is when I would probably get the most out of it. I find it far easier to write about exciting positive experiences than about complex upsetting ones. Invariably I need to talk about the painful experiences and get them into some kind of perspective before I commit them to paper. I think that this is because writing is a solitary occupation and it is quite uncomfortable to scrutinize your involvement in a less than successful situation without someone to support you. This is an area of my reflective practice that I am consciously trying to develop at the moment.

I find that to write effectively in my journal I like to be physically comfortable. I have a bath, get a cup of tea and then take myself upstairs where I will be guaranteed some peace and quiet. I like to sit at a desk, and write with a particularly nice fountain pen. These details seem irrelevant but I find them quite important to achieving the correct frame of mind. My journal is an A4 book, I write my description of a situation and relevant surrounding factors on the left-hand page and then write the reflection and analysis on the right-hand page. I find this particularly useful because I can then return to this right-hand page at any time in the future and continue to scribble ideas as my understanding of a situation develops. It fascinates me that I still refer to some incidents of long ago and can read new and different meanings into them. I believe that as I develop and grow as a person I learn more about myself and can understand more of my past behaviours as a result. Sometimes I write in my journal in smooth prose, at other times I just jot down key points and link the thoughts with lines and doodles. I am constantly amazed at how my ideas flow and how these ideas seem to develop as a result of this struggle to express them on paper. I personally find it much easier to reflect on my actions verbally than in a written form, but I value both methods, hence my perseverance with my journal.

As my skills of reflection develop, I find that I am increasingly reflecting in action as well as upon action. I am aware that whilst I am involved in a situation I am assessing the effectiveness of my interventions and often subtly changing how I do something as a result of this. This leads me into reflective conversations with colleagues who may also have been involved in the situation. I have found that there is a particular value in reflecting upon an incident as closely as possible to the event. Memories are clearer for the nuances of an interaction which can make all the difference to understanding why a situation evolved as it did. More often than not this is impossible due to pressure of work, however it is important to recognize the occasions when this opportunity does arise.

Some of my colleagues have reflective partners, that is one person whom they regularly reflect with. I find that I tend to discuss certain situations with particular people, but I do not reflect regularly with just one person. I have found it valuable to reflect with people inside and outside a particular situation. I am aware that the colleagues that I do reflect with have particular characteristics in common. They are all people whom I respect as practitioners, and whose opinion I value. It is important that I feel safe, to express my thoughts and ideas without fear of judgment so that I can be myself and truly share my thoughts, feelings, and reactions.

I probably do not reflect formally as regularly as I would like, however I suspect that this could always be the case regardless of the time you devoted to it. I think that just as it is important to recognize when one should reflect it is also vital to identify when enough is enough. It is important not to become so introspective that one is paralysed into inactivity.

This chapter is a very personal account of the meaning of reflection to one person. I hope that it encourages some of you to have a go. One of the best things about reflection is that you will always learn something that will enhance your clinical practice, no matter how much of a novice you may be. Learning about reflection has enabled me to transform my nursing practice. This transformation has taken place gradually over a period of years as I have learnt more about nursing and myself. One of the most valuable things that I have gained from this process is the ability to express my thoughts about nursing, and to share them with others. I can express my thoughts more clearly because I have learnt how to recognize the different types of knowledge that go together to make up my clinical practice. I have also learnt ways of analysing that knowledge, and the importance of a balance between rational and intuitive thought. I now recognize the value of an intuitive way of thinking about my practice. Intuitive thought involves holistic perception, imagination and creativity, these are the very cornerstones of inspired nursing care.

What follows is an exemplar from my journal. On the right hand page is my description of the situation and on the left hand page my analysis and reflection. For clarity the relevant entries have been numbered.

Reflection and analysis

(1)   I picked up early warning signals. I would not have been able to do this if I had not known Julie's capabilities so well.

(2)   This is contextual information. It is important to really know great detail of a patient's situation so that you can identify and interpret problems from their perspective. We were all aware that David had been through an enormous ordeal but was getting to the end of his energy that he could use to rise to each new challenge.

(3)   I believe that this demonstrates skill in acquiring information in a busy clinical environment in an almost imperceptible way. I had not been aware of paying that much attention to David and Julie as they had passed me, I had been on a ward round at the time. The relevance of this information only occurred to me afterwards, as I walked towards the room. I was already exploring potential problems.

(4)   I instantly recognized the seriousness of the problem. Julie did not volunteer much information, she wanted me to reach my own conclusions, and to assess the problem independently.

(5)   David had had PCA running since his admission. He was fully involved in his pain management. This in itself was the result of teamwork and a consistency of approach to this problem by the nursing and two medical teams who were involved in his care.

(6)   I assessed the problem rapidly, recognizing options. I was using pharmacological knowledge and previous experience of the effectiveness of these drugs in practice. Simple solutions could have been to persuade him to have either the suppository or injection on the basis that these were what the doctor had prescribed. I could have convinced David that the pain was not as severe as he thought. It would soon settle. I could have persuaded him that the pain must be getting less because he had already had a generous amount of morphine. None of these options were considered because of my belief of what nursing is and the purpose of nursing action.

I reassured David that the sensations were a direct result of the surgery that he had just undergone, whilst checking that the bandage was not too tight. I explained the tightness as the result of the wound being drawn together. This again demonstrates the value I place on the patient understanding what is happening and why. I thought that David may have associated the pain with something going wrong. I knew that knowledge was vital to David in terms of his coping strategy. David was

My exemplar

'Mid morning on a busy early shift one of the team leaders (Julie) came up to me and asked for my assistance with one of her patients. I was instantly alarmed because her face was tense and unsmiling.

(1)   Julie was an extremely experienced nurse who had worked on the ward for two years and rarely came across a clinical problem that she could not resolve. I soon realised that we were heading towards David's room.

David was one of Julie's primary patients, I knew him well as I was working in Julie's team at this time.

(2)   David was 25 years old, he had been on the ward for eight weeks with acute renal failure, and an ischaemic left leg with grossly infected wounds. David had had his leg amputated ten days ago, the wound had been left open because of the infection that was present at the time of the operation. David had recently completed undergraduate studies, and had travelled extensively independently prior to his illness.

He was terrified by the lack of apparent control that he now had over his life, his body and his future. David's coping strategy was to find out as much as possible about his condition. He asked questions constantly. David was weak and vulnerable, physically and emotionally. He did not want to shave or wash or cut his hair, he looked like an old man. It was evident to all that David was getting to the end of his ability to cope with what he was going through.

On this particular morning David had been to theatre to have his amputation wound surgically closed. Usually a member of his family was with him constantly but when David went to theatre they took the opportunity to have a break from hospital life.

Julie had escorted David back from the recovery department 15 minutes earlier. I noticed that he looked settled when they went past me in the corridor.

(3)   My mind raced as we walked towards David's room. Julie told me that David was in 'a complete state'. There was no time to get further details from Julie as she needed to get back to David.

(4)   We walked into his room and I saw David lying totally motionless on his bed. His face was grey and looked totally expressionless, his eyes looked blank.

I knelt down to speak to David and rested my hand upon his. I asked him what was the matter and he told me he had been woken by sudden severe pain, that his leg hurt him more than he could bear. He told me that his leg felt tight and throbbing, with shooting pains from where he felt the wound was. I asked him at what level his pain was at on his scoring system, he told me it was 5, worst imaginable pain.

Reflection and analysis *cont.*

so weak and vulnerable it would have been all too easy to have taken advantage of this and chosen a simple solution to his problem whilst overriding his wishes by simply not recognizing them. Even rolling over in bed for a suppository was more than he could contemplate. An IM injection was perceived as just one more pain to add to all the others he already had. This is evidence that my beliefs regarding the meaning of nursing are supported by my clinical practice.

My actions support my beliefs about nursing here, even though David is in distress I recognize the importance of discovering what his problem is. Not Julie's interpretation of his problem. I had confidence in my clinical skills to be able to extract the relevant information from David swiftly and accurately. Despite feeling wretched David gave me very specific information. I believe that this is due to the emphasis that we had all placed on David assessing his own pain since his admission. If he had not developed this skill it would have been impossible for him to have responded to my question in such an accurate manner when in distress.

(7)   Julie and I both knew that our surgeons even if they had been readily available did not have the specific knowledge of pain relief that was needed. We recognized that we had sufficient knowledge and experience to know what to do. This shows I value my nursing knowledge and experience and recognize that I have a complementary role to the medical staff. I know my own limitations and those of the staff that I regularly work with. I accepted David's definition of the problem whilst recognizing the surrounding factors. It also reveals my belief in the influence of the mind over the body, the interdependence of the two. Again we come back to the meaning that this pain holds for David.

This decision was based upon prior knowledge and experience of giving intravenous opiates. I was aware of the implications of my actions, not just in a practical sense but in a medicolegal sense too. I was aware as I made my decision that I had backup in the room should David's respiratory function be compromised as a result of my action. We also had Naloxone in the room. The decision was not taken lightly but in my assessment of the situation I could see no alternative to relieve David's distress.

(8)   I think my course of action demonstrated the commitment that I had to help him. It was the only action that I could see to take that would be acceptable to both of us. David trusted me and had faith in me that I would be able to help him. In view of the nature of our relationship I recognized that immediate action was called for.

My exemplar *cont.*

(5)   I noticed that he had a cannula in his arm with patient controlled analgesia in progress, he said that he had as much as the program would allow. I looked at the pump and saw that this was correct, he had received 8 mg of morphine intravenously in the last hour. We discussed other options, he was prescribed Diclofenac as a suppository or intramuscular injection. David refused both of these options as he said that he could not move and could not face any more needles. He looked directly at me and said quietly, "please no more, just no more anything".

(6)   Julie and I looked at each other, this was where she had been prior to getting me. We both realized that something needed to be done quickly. All our doctors were in theatre, it would take too long to get any of them up to the ward.

(7)   I realized that David was obviously in a great deal of pain, but knowing him also recognized that extreme anxiety was exacerbating his pain and decreasing his ability to cope with it. I understood that David was terrified that his leg wound might still not heal and realized that he also knew that the next option would be a much higher level of amputation, at hip level. David did not mention the absence of his mother, but I am sure that this added to his distress.

I decided that the only way to relieve David's pain was to give him morphine until he felt the pain was bearable.

(8)   I explained to David that I would give him a bolus injection of his morphine solution from his PCA [patient controlled analgesia] syringe until he felt comfortable. As I explained this to David I saw Julie in my peripheral vision and noticed a slight inclination of her head.

(9)   She knew that what I was doing was unusual but I thought/hoped that she approved. It seemed inappropriate to discuss the situation at that moment.

As I took the syringe from the pump I explained to David that the analgesia in the syringe was morphine, one of the most powerful painkilling drugs in existence. I knew that David always appreciated information and it seemed natural to continue talking.

(10)   As I did I was aware that my voice was low, but audible and the tone was level and well modulated. I spoke slowly, steadily and continuously, giving David something to focus on other than his perception of his situation.

I spoke of the passage of the morphine from the syringe through the fine plastic tube into the vein in his arm and into his blood stream. I explained that the morphine would swiftly pass through his body to arrive at the site of his pain. At this point I asked David to imagine the morphine at his wound site counteracting the pain, which was getting less and less as each moment

Reflection and analysis *cont.*

(9)   I could not discuss the reasoning behind my action with Julie at that moment as it would have changed the focus within the room from David's needs to our professional needs. This also demonstrates the interdependence that grows with close team work. I realized that Julie and I had very similar thoughts regarding the meaning of nursing. I also knew that this was my decision and that I alone was accountable for the ramifications that may stem from my action. I was aware that I was bending if not breaking the rules by not discussing my action with the medical staff beforehand. This courage to take risks with my clinical practice has grown as a result of my own professional confidence from working in one clinical area for five years. I have a good working relationship with my medical colleagues and we had often had difficult moments in the past in relation to David's pain control. I was not doing anything that we had not contemplated doing in the past.

(10)   The way in which I administered this bolus injection of morphine was congruent with my beliefs of the value of non pharmacological approaches to pain relief. I was trying to help David get some sense of control over his situation. To help him to think in a more positive way, hence the visualization and description of my actions. I needed to give David something to focus upon other than how bad his pain was. I knew my description of the action of the morphine was not pharmacologically correct but I wanted to describe it in a graphic way that would help David in his fight to gain control over his pain. The breathing exercise was another terribly conscious action on my part to help David to relax because I was sure that his tension and fear were exacerbating his experience of pain.

(11)   I hope that my skills were used in a subtle way, and integrated as a whole rather than appearing as a pot pourri of dissociated actions. Julie confirmed afterwards that it had appeared a subtle combination of skills. I don't know if I have ever wanted to make a difference to anyone's situation quite this badly before. I was amazed at the depth of my concentration upon David. It really mattered to me that I help David to cope with what he was going through. I'm sure my commitment helped, my presence at his bedside willing him to find the strength.

(12)   When I realized that David was relaxing, that his pain was fading, I felt totally elated. As I mentally withdrew from the situation I was extremely surprised that such a short space of time had passed and that he had received such a small dose of morphine. On analysis it is very difficult to say which aspect of my actions had the most influence over David, however the power of the combination of strategies used is indisputable.

My exemplar *cont.*

passed as more and more painkiller arrived continuously in his blood stream.

I asked David to feel the pain ebbing away, with each breath he was breathing the pain out of his body. I asked him to focus on the pain leaving his body, to breathe slowly and deeply and breathe the pain away.

(11)   Whilst doing this I was aware of very very slowly pressing the plunger of the syringe. My other hand remained over David's, I kept my finger on his pulse so that I could assess his reaction to the drug I was giving him. I was oblivious to anything beyond the confines of David and myself. My concentration upon him, his situation, and his pain was total.

I was unaware of the passage of time. Eventually David began to relax his eyes, from being unfocused, met mine. His face looked less tense and his breathing took on a regular rate of ten breaths per minute, his pulse rate was 64. I lowered my voice further and then stopped talking and just watched David, he appeared to have fallen asleep.

(12)   At this point I looked at my watch and realized that I had only been in the room seven minutes. It had felt like hours. It had seemed as if David had been in pain for a long, long time, however less than ten minutes had passed from where David had suddenly woken up with the severe pain and Julie had come to get help. I looked at the syringe in my hand. David had received 1 mg of morphine since I removed the syringe from the pump.'

References

Carper, B. (1978) Fundamental patterns of knowing in nursing. *Advances in Nursing Science*, **1**(1), 13–23.

Dewey, J. (1933) *How We Think*. D.C. Heath, Boston.

Jarvis, P. (1987) *Adult Learning in the Social Context*, Croom Helm, London.

McKee, C. (1991) Breaking the mould. In *Nursing as Therapy*, McMahon, R. & Pearson, A. Chapman & Hall, London.

Paterson, G. & Zderad, L.T. (1976) *Humanistic Nursing*. John Wiley & Sons Inc., New York.

Schön, D. (1983), *The Reflective Practitioner*. Basic Books, Harper Collins, San Francisco.

Schön, D. (1987), *Educating the Reflective Practitioner*. Jossey-Bass, San Francisco.

Street, A. (1990) *Nursing Practice: High hard ground, messy swamps and the pathways in between*. Deakin University Press, Geelong.

Chapter 7
The Personal Side of Reflection

Introduction

This chapter explores the role reflection can play in enabling health care professionals to meet the demands of dying patients and families, an aspect of practice which is frequently identified as difficult and stressful (Bailey & Clarke (1989), Hingley & Cooper (1986), Hockley (1989), Vachon (1987)). Most of the discussion will be drawn from our experience with qualified health care professionals undertaking the Diploma in Higher Education in Palliative Care currently offered by Oxford Brookes University in partnership with Sir Michael Sobell House, Oxford. In this context we have found that reflection is valuable in enabling students to recognize and understand the interface between personal and professional experience and how this influences their response to dying patients, their families and friends.

Caring for dying patients and their families

Most nurses are regularly exposed to dying patients and their families (Field (1989), Webber (1989)) and yet this aspect of care continues to raise anxieties (Bailey & Clarke, 1989). Many factors interact within this experience, most importantly the personality and abilities of an individual and the environment in which he or she is working (Hingley & Cooper (1986), Vachon (1987)), Bailey and Clarke (1989). For example, Vachon (1987) found that the work environment, an individual's occupational role and patient and family variables were perceived as causing stress in relation to caring for a dying patient and their family.

Furthermore, Vachon (1987) argues that personal beliefs can interface with these professional factors, either consciously or unconsciously. For example, Vachon & Pakes (1984) found such beliefs to include always being patient and understanding; being beyond emotions such as depression, anger, frustration and despair; being able to relate equally well to all patients and families; being capable of separating the stresses of their personal and professional lives. Personal beliefs such as these are often deeply embedded in cultural patterns (Vachon, 1987) and it is likely that health care professionals are influenced in this way through socialization into the community they live and work in (Field, 1989).

In a similar way, there are many conscious and unconscious factors and beliefs which drive an individual's motivation to work with dying patients and their families. For example, many nurses are motivated by the belief that their role is to enable a person to die 'peacefully and with dignity' (Webber, 1989). Vachon (1987) has found similar factors which include wanting to control illness, pain and death; wanting to be associated with a charismatic leader; responding to a religious or humanistic calling; and unconsciously wanting to work through previous personal experiences through working with people who are undergoing a similar experience.

This personal-professional interface can influence professional practice (Vachon, 1987) and where these beliefs are idealistic or unachievable, as described above (Vachon (1987), Vachon & Pakes (1984)), they may lead to the health carer becoming anxious and stressed and consequently detached from the situation that they are involved with, or overwhelmed by it (Hingley & Cooper, 1986).

This detachment from dying patients is often achieved by various physical and cognitive distancing techniques which prevent or limit any interaction with dying patients. For example, nurses' reluctance to respond to dying patients was demonstrated by Bowers (1975) who found that nurses took significantly more time to answer call bells rung by dying patients compared to other groups of patients. In addition, when with dying patients health care workers frequently employ tactics to control conversations, guiding the content towards safe topics such as physical care required and only responding to cues from the patient which are perceived as 'safe' (Macquire (1986), Webster (1981)).

Until recently, there have been few acknowledgements of interfacing personal and professional experiences within practice. Understanding this interface may enable nurses and other care professionals to gain insight into beliefs about and motivations for working in health care settings. An awareness of this personal-professional interface can therefore be seen as a key to working effectively with dying patients and their families. It is for this reason that we see reflection as a crucial tool in enabling students to explore this aspect of themselves in order to begin to address some of the demands that caring for dying patients inevitably brings. While there are potential benefits in this approach to learning, it is nevertheless an approach that is very personal and can be difficult, and sometimes, painful.

Understanding who we are as people

As individuals we have the ability to stand back and look at ourselves. Mead (1934) attaches this activity as part of reflexive ability, i.e. the self as an object to itself. Mead perceives this ability as an essential component of the self. In other words, the self (i.e. the I, me) cannot exist without the ability to look at itself. However, the issue is not so much about whether we have the ability to understand ourselves, but rather how we use the information available to us to do so. Most of the information that we base our understanding of ourselves on, comes from three main sources: other people's perceptions of us, observing our thoughts and feelings, and observing our behaviour (Hampson, 1988). Of these three sources the major influence seems to be others' perceptions of us (Bem (1972), Hampson (1988), Mead (1934)).

It would seem that, for the most part, we gain knowledge about ourselves from other people's knowledge and perceptions of us. We therefore have a body of self knowledge that we feel comfortable with and which seems reasonable to other people. However, this knowledge is not the product of self examination and may therefore not be accurate (Hampson, 1988). Bem (1972) goes further and suggests that opinions about oneself are based on behaviours (as seen by others), rather than on the true nature of ourselves.

Bem (1972) stresses that this tendency to base our self knowledge on other people's perceptions of us only exists when we have few cues from our internal self. If we are able to increase information about ourselves by reflecting on our thoughts, feelings and behaviour, then it is likely that self knowledge would arise from within ourselves, rather than information gained from other sources. This is one of the strengths that reflection has to offer – helping us know ourselves. It encourages the development of the ability to examine actions, thoughts and feelings.

This potential for increased self-awareness does not come without a price. If the information gained about ourselves from others is likely to be inaccurate, then as we find out about ourselves, from our internal self, we are likely to experience a disparity between what we thought of ourselves previously and what the new information from our internal self is telling us about the nature of oneself. In addition, we may start to find out things about ourself which we were previously unaware of, or have unconsciously buried, and we may have to form a completely new view of our ideal self to match the new information that we have about ourselves. It is therefore not surprising that this process of finding out about oneself can be very powerful as well as painful.

Our experiences of using reflection within the Diploma in Higher Education in Palliative Care

Reflection is used within this course as a tool to enable students to develop self-awareness and critical inquiry. Students are encouraged to use a diary to record their thoughts and feelings about their experiences in clinical practice. It is hoped that themes will emerge from this record which will then guide students to further exploration through reading and analysis. The starting point to this process is often a critical incident, for example an experience with a patient or relative or a member of staff – a 'star' moment – something that makes an impression on the student. For instance, in the exemplar below, the starting point was a conversation with a patient. A summarized form of this incident and any first thoughts about it are presented in a learning contract as emerging evidence of learning. The mentor will then prompt and guide the student's further investigation through the use of critical questions in the learning contract. The student can then respond to these comments and in this way a dialogue and interaction can develop between student and mentor.

Using reflection in this way has exposed us to many experiences. We have seen many powerful and salient examples of practice in which the personal and professional experiences have merged. These examples capture palliative care practice at its very best. Equally, we have come across students who experience considerable difficulties in trying to use this approach to learning. Some of this difficulty centres around the language in which this is expressed (what is a learning contract, reflection?) but much of it is related to past experiences. For instance, those students who have previously believed that to be professional in your approach to care means that you are detached personally have found using reflection fundamentally difficult since they are now being encouraged to look at themselves. Furthermore, reflection exposes personal beliefs, motivations and vulnerabilities. Recording and expressing experiences and feelings in writing makes explicit an individual's reaction to these things and this can be both a painful and powerful experience. The following exemplar highlights many of these points.

June is an experienced palliative care nurse working in an acute hospital. She had been called to see a patient, Molly, on a busy acute ward. Molly was a young mother, had been in hospital for a little while and had recently had some chemotherapy. Molly had told the ward sister she wanted to go home.Concerned about this, the sister had asked June to visit Molly that day. When she arrived on the ward June reviewed

Molly's treatment, suggested some changes, and then went into Molly's room. This is June's reflection of that interaction:

> 'I went into Molly's room and started to ask her why she wanted to go home. She just said that was all she wanted. I asked her if she had thought how her mother would cope. She withdrew from communications, the eye to eye contact was gone. She shrank down into her bed and completely avoided any contact with me. I sat very quietly and looking at this tiny emaciated girl blending into the whiteness of the pillow ... I was overwhelmed with sadness at my total inability to have communicated and helped her. I felt the tears (run) down my face and I must have muttered "Oh Molly, this must be really awful for you, how on earth can I help you?". Her tiny hand came from under the covers and her hand clasped mine as she gave me eye contact and started to cry. We cried together for five minutes and then we sat in silence for five minutes. Then Molly communicated like she has never done before.
>
> She told me how frightened she was of dying and leaving her family, especially her children and the two men who have meant the most to her – her ex-husband and the man she was now living with. We discussed where she would best feel most supported as regards her fears and she admitted that the hospital ward was best. We then discussed personalizing her room and that we would be able to do that. She went very tired and I left her.'

When June went back to check Molly later that day she found her chatting amicably with her mother with her quilt from home on the bed and her soft toys all around the room and photographs of her children on the side. June and her mother had agreed that she would stay in hospital until she died.

When reflecting on what this incident had taught her, June highlighted two themes. Firstly, the importance of personal experience within her role as a nurse, particularly the ability to use her feelings in her care: 'I learnt such a lot about not totally suppressing my feelings', and secondly, the importance of seeing caring as a two way process 'they still have pride and want to feel they can still give too'.

Two key questions are raised for us by such powerful experiences:

- How appropriate is this approach to learning, since there is no way of knowing what reflection is going to unearth for the individual?
- What kind and level of support is required for the use of reflection? For example, June was able to draw support from a close working relationship with an interdisciplinary team and mentor. How would she have felt and coped without this support?

From our limited experience, we have found that adequate support is crucial in the process of reflection. It can mitigate the stress caused by changing and disparate self perceptions, in the same way that it can minimise the anxiety and disruption caused by stressful life events (Vachon, 1987; Littlewood, 1992; Osterweis *et al.*, 1984).

Within the Diploma in Higher Education in Palliative Care we have provided a formalized support structure primarily through mentors and professional tutors. Additional support is available from student counsellors outside the course team and informal support from other students and peers.

Mentors have a key role in this support structure. Students are asked to choose their mentor and we suggest they choose someone they can trust to receive negative and positive feedback from. Wherever possible, this mentor should work in the student's practice area and have palliative care expertise. Sometimes students have chosen two mentors so that they have someone in their clinical area as their first mentor (someone they trust) and someone with palliative care experience as a second mentor (such as a tutor, lecturer-practitioner or Macmillan nurse).

We recommend that students have access to a mentor with palliative care expertise for two main reasons. Firstly, this expertise enables students to debate palliative care issues in depth and in relation to their own practice setting. Secondly, the professional issues raised in learning contracts, such as the impact of dying on family relationships, could be potentially painful to the mentor as well as to the student exploring such issues. By recommending experience in the subject area that we are exploring we are minimizing the chance that mentors will be confronted by these potentially painful issues for the first time when reading the student's contract.

However, what cannot be avoided or minimised is the powerful impact that reflection can have in a written format. In part, this is a result of students being immersed in the practice situations they are writing about and expressing their experiences in a very personal way. It is also very difficult to avoid the content of a written discussion. For many mentors and students this sharing of written reflection has been a moving experience and has highlighted the intricate nature of clinical practice.

The implication of this is that support does not stop with the provision of mentors – the mentors need preparation and support. Equally, module leaders and professional tutors who have the remit for supporting students and mentors also need support. Sometimes this can be through reflection as a support strategy *per se* and sometimes through the quality of the relationship between the individuals involved.

It is therefore important to consider the factors which may influence the quality of relationship between a student and those supporting her/him. It is likely that certain attributes in the supporter (whether mentor or professional tutor), will help the student feel comfortable and able to develop individual understanding of themselves at a pace, and depth, that they feel happy with. Some of these attributes will be common to any interpersonal relationship, but, it is important to stress, that the relationship that we encourage between student and supporter is not viewed as counselling or therapy. Where this is thought to be necessary we would refer the student to professional help available through the student counselling services.

With these limits in mind, it is possible to draw on the literature to elicit what helps in the development of a supportive relationship. Rogers (1951) feels that the key element to any interactions of this kind is the quality of the relationship (rather than what exactly is said). This view is supported by a number of studies, for example, those looking at the efficacy of bereavement support (Osterweis *et al.*, 1984). This quality in a relationship can be fostered by genuineness, warmth and respect, and empathetic understanding (Nelson-Jones, 1982). It is probable that out of these three attributes, empathy is the central key. Fiedler (1950) describes this as 'to understand, to communicate with, and maintain rapport with' (p. 444).

These supportive qualities need to be available to students on an ongoing basis, since any challenge to an individual's self concept will take time to assimilate and incorporate. The support provided within a mentoring relationship may prevent deflecting strategies such as physical or cognitive avoidance being employed or maintained. These deflecting strategies are used to block new information being incor- porated into the internal view of the self, in order that values about the self can be maintained. Recently, Newell (1992) highlighted this possi- bility as a potential weakness of reflection, asserting the effect of memory and anxiety on accurate recall. He argues that as reflection depends on memory, then reflection can be biased by individual cue selection. Newell (1992) develops his argument by looking at the effect that stress has on the ability to encode information for recall. He suggests that reflection on difficult personal interactions (such as breaking bad news) may be affected by the level of stress that this arouses. The result may be that various defences are utilised to avoid this stress in the future, thereby avoiding the chance to reflect on this situation and develop appropriate skills to manage it.

Conclusion: implications of using reflection

While this chapter has raised some potential difficulties that reflection may evoke, overall our experience of reflection has been positive. We have seen many examples of the advantages that reflection can offer, such as the ability to make practice issues more explicit and the process for interfacing personal and professional experiences within practice. However, it is clear that the use of reflection has the potential to expose vulnerabilities and for some, threaten deep seated coping mechanisms.

The key issues that reflection raises for us centre on two areas: the importance of support, and the moral issue of whether we should be encouraging students to expose themselves without ever really knowing what an individual's past experiences had been. We also have concern for those mentors who may feel overwhelmed by some of the reflections raised by the students. In our evaluation of the course at the end of the first year, it was noteworthy that student and mentor relationships were strengthened, and that this relationship had, for most students and mentors, become mutually supportive.

Reflecting on the period that we have been supporting students, we have found it helpful to be clear about where responsibilities lay and to keep things in perspective. For instance, we needed to remind ourselves that reflection is a process. In this process we have a responsibility to support students and mentors and provide them with any resources needed but we cannot take away any distress raised by reflection. To do so would be to undermine the students' experience and maybe inhibit them from moving on through the process. Once the initial difficulty of grappling with reflection and learning contracts has passed, many students find reflection liberating, enabling them to be in touch with their feelings when caring for others. The recognition that it is alright to 'feel' whilst caring is often the first step in identifying motives for being involved with patients and families and developing effective skills required for that involvement.

From our experience of using reflection within a palliative care course, we can summarize the implications as follows:

- Reflection offers a powerful way to explore the interface between personal and professional experiences in practice. It provides a process for understanding how our personal lives mediate our responses to the demands made in our professional lives. This understanding has the potential to reduce the stress experienced in our professional lives.
- Support is an essential component of using this approach. It is important to reiterate that this does not stop with the provision of mentors but extends to everyone encouraging its use.
- There may be certain characteristics within this support that enable reflection to be honest and searching. It is likely that the quality of the interaction is more important than what is said and that this quality can be fostered by genuineness, warmth, respect and understanding.
- Reflection and support should not be seen as counselling or therapy.

Professional support should be available when the issues raised by reflection are overwhelming.

- Time needs to be spent explaining reflection throughout the course. This is because reflection has a language of its own and needs to be demystified. In our experience students ask for clear frameworks to help them go about using reflection – how to set out a reflective journal, how to present reflection in learning contracts. These frameworks can be helpful while students are developing their own personal style of reflection.
- The number of people involved in supporting students makes this approach to learning a potentially costly way of delivering a course. However, this commitment has potential benefits such as providing opportunities for care to be delivered by sensitive practitioners who may not be afraid to question their practice and motives for working in palliative care.

References

Bailey, R. & Clarke, M. (1989) *Stress and Coping in Nursing*. Chapman & Hall, London.

Bem, D.J. (1972) Self-Perception Theory. In Berkowitz, L. (Ed.) *Advances in Experimental Social Psychology*, Vol. 6, pp. 1–62. Academic Press, New York.

Bowers, M. (1975) *Counselling the Dying*. Jarson Aronson, New York.

Fiedler, F.E. (1950) The concept of an ideal therapeutic relationship. *Journal of Consulting Psychology*, **14**, 444.

Field, D. (1989) *Nursing The Dying*, Tavistock/Routledge, London.

Hampson, S.E. (1988) *The Construction of Personality*, Routledge, London.

Hingley, P. & Cooper, C. (1986) *Stress and the Nurse Manager*, Wiley and Sons, Chichester.

Hockley, J. (1989) Caring for the dying in acute hospitals. *Nursing Times*, **85**, No 39, 47–50.

Littlewood, J. (1992) *Aspects of Grief*. Tavistock/Routledge, Blackwells, London.

Macquire, P. (1986) Barriers to psychological care of the dying. *British Medical Journal*, **291**, 1711–13.

Mead, G.H. (1934). *Mind, Self and Society*. University of Chicago Press, Chicago.

Nelson-Jones, R. (1982) *The Theory and Practice of Counselling Psychology*. Cassell Educational Ltd, London.

Newell, R. (1992). Anxiety, accuracy and reflection: the limits of professional development. *Journal of Advanced Nursing*, **17** (11), 1326–33.

Osterweis, M., Solomon, N. and Green, M. (1984) *Bereavement Reactions, Consequences and Care*. National Academy Press, Washington D.C.

Rogers, C.R. (1951) *Client Centred Therapy*. Houghton Mifflin, Boston.

Sherr, L. (1989) *Death, Dying and Bereavement*. Blackwell Scientific Publications, Oxford.

Vachon, M.L.S. & Pakes, E.H. (1984) Staff stress in the care of the critically ill and dying child. In Wass, H. & Corr, C.A. (Eds) *Childhood and Death*. Hemisphere Publishers, Washington D.C.

Vachon, M.L.S. (1978) Motivation & stress experiences by staff working with the terminally ill. *Death Education*, **2**, 113–22.

Vachon, M.L.S. (1987) *Occupational Stress In The Care of the Critically Ill, the Dying and the Bereaved.* Hemisphere Publishers, Washington D.C.

Webber, J. (1989) *The effects of an educational course on problems identified by nurses caring for patients with advanced cancer.* MSc dissertation, University of London.

Webster, M. (1981) Communicating with dying patients. *Nursing Times*, 4 June, **88**, 999–1002.

Chapter 8
Guided Reflection

Introduction

Guided reflection is a combination of techniques intended to enable practitioners to reflect on their professional work experiences in order to become increasingly effective. This method was introduced to practitioners at Burford Community Hospital in 1989 within a collaborative research study which aimed to identify and understand the essential aspects of defined therapeutic work and factors that limited therapeutic potential (Johns, 1993).

A central theme within the work is the concept of *guided* reflection, enabling practitioners to utilise and learn through reflection on experiences, in a structured and supported way.

The process of guided reflection

Reflection is a mirror to practice. Through reflection, practitioners can come to see themselves in the context of their practices and develop the essential skills and values associated, which characterize therapeutic work (Johns, 1993). By therapeutic I mean actions carried out with the intention of benefiting the patient/family. Reflection can be arduous and painful at times. Evidence from the research study and evaluation of reflective practice modules at Luton College suggests that reflection is a profoundly difficult thing to do without expert guidance and support.

Consider a number of potential questions that face the prospective reflective practitioner.

- What is reflection?
- How do you do it?
- How do you know if you are doing it?
- Am I doing it properly?
- Which of my experiences should I reflect on?

- How do I learn through reflection?
- How do I become aware of the factors that limit my therapeutic and reflective potential?
- Who will support me when things get tough?

The description of reflection offered in other chapters of this book considers the question 'what is reflection?' to some extent. Yet knowing this does not necessarily enable the practitioners to use reflection in a meaningful way in practice. The literature on becoming a reflective practitioner is limited in answering these questions beyond theoretical accounts. For example – knowing the essential learning domains to becoming an effective practitioner does not enable the practitioner to become skilled. However they do enable the practitioner to consider her own performance in relation to these domains and hence they offer a focus for reflection.

Consider an example where a district nurse is unable to assert with a certain GP the use of a different bladder wash out which she knows will be more effective. She feels unable to fulfil her perceived role as her patient's advocate and as a consequence her patient suffers unnecessary blockage and leakage of his catheter and thus becomes increasingly depressed.

One solution to this problem could be to undertake an assertiveness training course. The nurse may come to understand the nature of assertiveness and may even be able to enact her difficulty with the general practitioner in role play situations. Yet when she returns to practice, even though she is now informed she is frequently unable to transfer the learning from the classroom into practice. The reality is that she has been socialized into a subordinate role in relation to doctors which has become a barrier to learning. Such barriers are not so easily overcome. However, by reflecting on a series of similar experiences with this doctor over time, the district nurse may eventually learn to become more assertive.

This example highlights a need for guidance and support for the reflective practitioner. With guidance the district nurse can be helped to understand the nature of the problem, and to develop strategies to overcome this barrier. Guidance also offers support. The failure to be assertive may be deeply distressing to the district nurse, and her attempts to overcome this problem are likely to make her feel vulnerable and anxious.

There are three elements to guided reflection:

(1) Using the Model of Structured Reflection.
(2) Supervision.
(3) Diary Structure.

Model of structured reflection

The model (Fig. 8.1) consists of a series of questions which aim to tune the practitioner into her experience in a structured and meaningful way. It emerged as a natural sequence through which practitioners explored their experiences in supervision.

Illustrated on pages 113–18 is an example of using the model shown in Fig. 8.1 in practice, interspersed with my comments.

Core question – What information do I need access to in order to learn through this experience?

Cue questions –

1.0 *Description of experience*
  .1 *Phenomenon* – Describe the 'here and now' experience.
  .2 *Causal* – What essential factors contributed to this experience?
  .3 *Context* – What are the significant background actors to this experience?
  .4 *Clarifying* – What are the key processes (for reflection) in this experience?

2.0 *Reflection*
  .1 What was I trying to achieve?
  .2 Why did I intervene as I did?
  .3 What were the consequences of my actions for:
    – Myself?
    – The patient/family?
    – For the people I work with?
  .4 How did I feel about this experience when it was happening?
  .5 How did the patient feel about it?
  .6 How do I know how the patient felt about it?

3.0 *Influencing factors*
  .1 What internal factors influenced my decision making?
  .2 What external factors influenced my decision making?
  .3 What sources of knowledge did/should have influenced my decision making?

4.0 Could I have dealt better with the situation?
  .1 What other choices did I have?
  .2 What would be the consequences of these choices?

5.0 *Learning*
  .1 How do I *now* feel about this experience?
  .2 How have I made sense of this experience in light of past experiences and future practice?
  .3 How has this experience changed my ways of knowing:
    – empirics?
    – aesthetics?
    – ethics?
    – personal?

Fig. 8.1 Model of structured reflection (Johns (1992) and Carper (1978)).

Description

Reflection always commences with a description of the 'here and now' of the experience. The description of experience extends to consider the factors that contribute to it within the context in which the experience takes place. An analogy would be dropping a stone into a pond. The splash is the here and now. The ripples moving out from the splash are the contributing factors, whilst the pond is the context of this experience.

Phenomenon [practitioner describing the experience]

'Rachel, the daughter of a patient (Mavis) burst into tears when I asked her how she was coping at home with Mavis. I immediately felt embarrassed and anxious about how I should respond. I asked Rachel to sit down in the staff room and made her some tea. I asked her if I could help her.

Fortunately the unit was not too busy. I asked the care assistant to take over helping Tom with his bath. Rachel then blurted out how she couldn't cope any more with caring for her mother at home and how it was destroying her marriage and making her ill.

After about ten minutes she said she mustn't take up any more of my time and that she was being silly. I said it was okay. She got up – wiped her tears with a tissue which I had offered her, said thank you, smiled and left. I wasn't sure how to follow it up.'

Causal

'Mavis was readmitted to the unit two days ago. She has been rude to staff and demanding help for things she used to do easily for herself. I had only been a primary nurse for three months and had only nursed Mavis on one previous admission.'

Context

'Mavis has been coming into hospital for two years now at regular intervals as a respite care patient. She lives at her daughter's home – Rachel and her husband Wilf. Mavis has always been a very "proper" lady although probably underneath the surface she always has some intolerance which she contains well. I think we've always got on well. Physically she is self-caring. Rachel and Wilf have always been friendly but have largely kept a distance from sharing their thoughts and feelings about caring and the future with Mavis.'

Clarifying [author's comments]

Clarifying intends to help the practitioner put the description of experience back together and to look at it as a whole, identifying the key processes manifest within the experience. It is useful to make a list of these processes even though the practitioner and supervisor may choose not to explore all of them.

Clarifying processes

(1) Prioritizing needs of patients/delegating work.
(2) My relationship with the relative and dealing with the feelings that emerge from this.
(3) Meeting the relative's needs/carers' needs.

Reflection

The reflection stage considers what the practitioner was trying to achieve, the reasons for acting as she did, and the consequences of her actions for the patient, herself, and others involved or affected by the experience.

What was I trying to achieve? [practitioner's comments]

'I wanted to comfort Rachel – to help her feel better. I also wanted her to tell me why she was so upset and see what the problems were for her.'

Why did I intervene as I did?

'I asked Rachel how she was coping almost as a routine remark – I didn't expect her to break down and cry. As I was her primary nurse I felt I needed to help her then. It also made me feel that I hadn't given enough attention to how Rachel and Wilf were keeping – in that sense I felt guilty. I just sat and listened to Rachel – giving her total attention – trying to tell her I had time to listen and cared for her.'

What were the consequences of my actions:

● *For myself*

'It made me realise I didn't know how Rachel had been coping at home or how she had been feeling. I had just taken it for granted that things were okay. I was also very unsure about how I could communicate with Rachel to give her the support she needed. This was influenced by my anxiety and not saying the wrong things – this was influenced by my guilt!'

● *For Rachel?*

'I hoped she thought that I had helped her. I think I did. I hope she thinks that I now know and that she can approach me again. I hope she thinks that the lid has now been taken off.'

- ## *For the people I work with?*

'I'm not sure at this moment. I looked through the notes – and there is nothing in the notes about Rachel and her husband Wilf – about their needs etc. in the assessment. I realize that's been an oversight.'

Parallel to this 'cognitive' element of reflection is an affective element concerned with recognising how the practitioner and others were feeling. This reflection aims to tune the nurse into her feelings and the feelings of the others in the experience. Caring is explicitly emotional work and as such the reflection aims to enable the practitioner to recognise and value her own feelings. Through this the practitioner can learn to show herself and the impact of herself on others in order to become therapeutic with her patients.

How did I feel about this experience when it was happening? [practitioner's comments]

'Awful – because I felt so guilty – I don't really know why I should have felt so guilty – because she was so upset and I asked her such a routine question. Dealing with her tears was also tough – I normally cope with patient's tears – but then I am normally more detached – with Rachel, it was so different – I really felt involved and didn't know how to respond for the best. I took a deep breath afterwards and realised I had been sweating.'

How did Rachel feel about it?

'Difficult to say. I can only repeat her words to me afterwards – she said thank you – smiled. She said she felt silly – I wonder if that's true – it must have been difficult for her to break down like that – she always seems such a controlled person.'

How do I know how the patient felt about it?

'Well, she was so tearful – it was easy to see she was upset. It was more difficult to tell afterwards. She appeared more relaxed, but seemed awkward. She also felt embarrassed afterwards.'

Influencing factors [author's comments]

The next stage is to consider the various factors and sources of knowledge that influenced the practitioner's decision making within the experience.

By internal factors I refer to factors within the practitioner, for example previous experience with similar patients, feelings of hostility towards the patient's family, intuition, feelings of subordination towards the doctor, etc. External factors include all professional and organisational factors, initially, it may be very difficult to see these. The practitioner needs to seek out relevant sources of knowledge that impact on this experience and consider how these become integrated in experience.

What factors/knowledge influenced my decisions and actions? [Practitioner explaining influencing factors]

(1) 'My original question was polite routine – I would say that to any relative of a respite care patient – I guess I wasn't thinking very much.

(2) On reflection I didn't know Rachel or Wilf very well – beyond superficial knowing – I didn't know how they managed at home. When I had talked to Mavis on the last admission she gave an impression that everything at home was fine. I didn't think to look beyond that – why should I – shouldn't I accept what the patient says is so?

(3) I haven't really read anything about respite care or the impact of caring on carers. I know I must do that now. It's surprising how we take things for granted. I know the model of nursing encourages me to look beyond the patient in the hospital bed – to see them as a member of their community etc – but it's easier said than done when you have never been encouraged to see patients that way before.

(4) I suppose my dubious communication skills played a part – because I don't really know if I helped or what!

(5) Because I was upset myself – that must have interfered with helping Rachel.'

Could I have dealt better with the situation? [author's comments]

'Hindsight is all very well – of course I could have. That sounds as if I am irritated with this – I'm not really – it's just anger at myself.'

This involves considering alternative actions and the consequences of those actions. Clearly, practitioners have a repertoire of interventions from which they choose when faced with complex clinical situations. Through the process of reflection, this repertoire is examined. Not only does the practitioner learn to use this repertoire more critically, she also begins to learn to extend it.

Considering alternative situations can then enable the nurse to be imaginative, creative and intuitive, whilst challenging her to extend the limits of her empirical knowledge.

What other choices did I have?

'At the time I only reacted – I couldn't think it out. So I suppose I had no other choices. On reflection it's so easy to look at myself and realise how awful it must have seemed. I think I did the right thing – to take Rachel away from Mavis into the staff room and help her to relax with a cup of tea and to listen to her. I wonder what Mavis felt about that – seeing Rachel cry like that. I never thought to talk with Mavis afterwards – she never mentioned it.

I know about Heron's interventions. Maybe if I had been more in control of myself I might have reflected-in-action about using the most appropriate interventions. For example, Rachel needed a lot of support, but she also needed a cathartic intervention – "I can see this hurts you Rachel".

But – I felt I didn't know her well enough to be like that with her. Not knowing her well enough limited my options. I was tempted to give her glib reassurance – "everything will be OK" – it surprised me how easy it is to just do that – I sensed that and was able to resist it – I guess that would only have been helping myself.'

What would have been the consequences of these other choices?

'If I had been cathartic I felt I would have got into even deeper water and wouldn't have coped with the situation at all. It's important that carers see you can cope with their distress – otherwise they will think you are stupid or incompetent ... wouldn't they? I don't know about that – that's an interesting thought.'

Learning [author's comments]

The final phase is to put the experience into a learning perspective. By focusing on how the practitioner is feeling now, it aims to enable the practitioner to express any residual feeling. It also links this experience with the past – inviting the practitioner to look back – and then link this to future practice. The aim is to enable the practitioner to see herself and her experiences in the context of historical and social processes.

How do I feel now about this experience?

'Still uncomfortable – I tried to talk to Jane (another primary nurse) about this experience but felt that she would think I was being silly. I know I failed and feel defensive about that. I need to talk to Rachel again about this – to show her I do care about her and Wilf – and to establish a more therapeutic relationship – I need to build up trust with Rachel.'

How have I made sense of this experience – in the light of past experiences and future practice?

It's quite frightening to read back through this reflection and realise how limited I am in my caring. This experience has really challenged who I am in relation to patients and relatives. I know that sounds ridiculous writing that – but I feel it's true.

The most important thing is establishing a relationship for the basis of caring. If I had known Rachel and had been really interested in her then I would have responded much better and coped much better. I know we have spoken previously about the mutuality of caring – now I can see this and appreciate it. The issue about writing in the notes is also important – just like the previous primary nurse I haven't written anything about Rachel and Wilf in the notes – that's important – what would have happened if an associate nurse had had this experience with Rachel? I did see Rachel again. I took her hand and asked her how she was feeling about our meeting three days earlier. She just looked at me – it was almost as if she was looking to see if I did care about her in my eyes. It was unnerving but I could now understand that. I just held her gaze, she smiled and said it had been helpful talking to me. I said to her that I have some time now to explore the future. She said "I'll spend a few minutes with Mother and then come and see you". I smiled back to her – still holding her hand and said "I'll have the kettle on".

That felt really great – and we were really able to explore the impact that caring had on her and some options for the future. I'm going to write about that later.

Difficulties in using the model and being reflective

The model, like most models, is not necessarily easy to use in practice. A problem with all models is their prescriptive attraction. As such, the risk is that practitioners will attempt to reduce their experiences to answering a series of questions that splinters the human encounter. The cue questions do not necessarily need specific answers. The practitioner should come to use the model in the way most helpful to themselves.

However, they may have difficulty in seeing beyond themselves and remain limited by their own narrow perceptions of themselves and their work. They may have difficulty identifying factors that limit their therapeutic potential because such factors have been so deeply engrained within them. They may have problems accessing relevant literature because they have no confidence themselves in being able to read, understand and apply such knowledge. They may also be convinced by professional knowledge rhetoric, that the only valued knowledge is research-based and consequently come to doubt or deny their own personal knowledge. As a result their sense of commitment to work has become blunted, preferring to exist in a blinkered, dogmatic and defended world rather than face the effort of curiosity, reflection and commitment; too scarred or burnt-out to care. The reality is that for many nurses reflection will be a tough and frustrating journey. As such I advocate that reflection should always be supervised or coached (Schön, 1987) in order to support the journey.

Supervision

Supervision as envisaged here, has its roots in psychotherapy and social work. It has been defined as an:

> 'Intensive, interpersonally focused, one to one relationship in which one person is designed to facilitate the development of therapeutic competence in the other person' (Loganbill, Hardy, & Delworth (1982) cited in Hawkins & Shohet (1989) p 41).

Whilst this definition emphasises a one-to-one relationship between a supervisor and the practitioners, supervision can also take place with groups of practitioners. However, this discussion will consider only individual supervision.

Who should the supervisor be?

I advocate that the supervisor should be the practitioner's line manager. This belief is based on my experience of working with primary nurses and district nurses where a key aspect of work has been to develop collegial relationships between the manager and practitioner.

Collegial relationships are based upon a mutual respect and understanding of each other's role. The role of the manager within primary and district nursing shifts from delegating tasks to devolving authority to individuals to manage a case load. As such, the role of the manager must shift from delegation to enabling and supporting to ensure primary nurses are effective. Yet, the reality is that many primary and district nurses are ill prepared for these roles. Supervision can enable them to succeed without undermining their prime responsibility for managing a caseload. I believe enabling practitioners to *succeed* in their roles is not an option for clinical leaders; it must be incumbent on them to achieve this work. Of course, the supervisor need *not* be the practitioner's manager. However, the benefits of this mutual process will be lost.

Contracting

Supervision relationships should always be framed within a personal contract between supervisor and practitioner that addresses issues such as control of input, confidentiality, regularity of meetings, expectations and responsibilities. Contracting sets the stage for a relationship built on trust; a climate of trust being essential to enable the practitioner to feel free to share her experiences without a fear of being judged.

Connecting

Within the supervision relationship, both supervisor and supervisee learn to relate to each other. This may require the supervisor having access to his or her own supervision. The key nature of the supervision relationship is connection. Belenky *et al.* (1986) note that:

> 'Since knowledge comes from experience the only way they can hope to understand another person's ideas is to try and share that experience that had led that person to form that idea.' (p. 113)

Connected teaching is receiving and accepting the student's thoughts and feelings towards the experience. As Belenky *et al.* further note: 'Connected teachers are believers, they trust their students' thinking and encourage them to expand it' (p. 227). This is not to say that the supervisor will not judge the practitioner's performance, it merely highlights that the prime role of supervision is to enable the practitioner to develop therapeutic effectiveness rather than a form of social or quality control. If the practitioner senses being judged or manipulated then she will be unlikely to share significant experiences in supervision.

'Connecting' also role models how the practitioner might be with her own patients. This is realising and exploiting the concept of a parallel process as a learning milieu (Johns, 1993). By this I refer to the aspects of the practitioner–patient relationship which are recreated within the supervisor–practitioner relationship. For example how the practitioner sees the patient – 'who is this person?', 'what are their needs?', 'how are they feeling?', 'how do they make me feel?' 'how can I help them?'

Moreover, many of the intervention techniques used by the practitioner are made explicit and role modelled for the practitioner to consider in working with patients.

Focus for reflection

What experiences the practitioner chooses to share is determined by herself. This control of input encourages the practitioner to take responsibility for her work, both in practice and in supervision, and is crucial for psychological safety. Using a model of structured reflection (see Fig. 8.1) enables the practitioner to reflect prior to the session thereby utilizing supervision time for more critical reflection.

Brookfield (1987) notes:

'there is always some "trigger" for reflection. Some unexpected happening prompts a sense of inner discomfort and perplexity' (p. 26).

Dewey (1933) writes of how reflection arises out of situations of doubt and perplexity and prompts action towards resolving the doubt. From my own experience I feel it is important to strike a balance at the outset between reflecting on problematic experiences and satisfying experiences, although practitioners tend to focus naturally on stressful experiences. The danger of focusing on only problematic experiences is that it gives the practitioner feedback that they are indeed problematic and may reinforce their own doubts about their ability and ensuing self-esteem.

Without doubt, much of nursing work involves working with people in intimate, emotional and often distressing aspects of care. I expect most nurses can remember saying to other people something like:

'I looked after this lady today, she died. I felt so upset because I felt so close to her and her daughter. The daughter just cried and cried. I just cried as well but I felt awful because I didn't know how to help her and I should be able to cope better than I did.'

Nurses may find it difficult to think about such experiences beyond a mere description of the events. It is difficult to think rationally on experiences when experiencing strong emotions such as anger, frustration or sadness about an event. The natural inclination is to attempt to rationalize or repress these emotions in an attempt to limit the distress or anxiety associated with the experience. This may be particularly true for nurses who have been socialized into defence systems that discourage the sharing of feelings behind the ubiquitous facade 'that good nurses cope'. Marshall (1980) reminds us, from her review of the stress literature on nursing, that nurses generally cope by avoiding situations that cause them anxiety. The need to reduce anxiety is a powerful motivator for the decisions and subsequent actions that nurses take in work situations. Hence if a situation causes the nurse anxiety, she is likely to react by avoiding reflecting about that situation. This apparent contradiction reflects the need for awareness, or intelligence as Fay (1987) calls this, to confront this avoidance.

In general nurses seem to find an oral account of experiences fairly easy to articulate, but find writing an account of the experience problematic. It is almost as if nurses begin to discount their experiences as insignificant, finding it difficult to value their own experiences and hence write about them. Trying to understand this phenomenon has left me with the impression that nurses have been socialized to devalue what they do, in helping patients with their complex psychological and physical needs. This discounting becomes very visible in research that highlights how 'emotional work' (James, 1989) and 'body work' (Lawler, 1991) with patients is highly skilled, yet perceived as largely unskilled, invisible and unvalued, and hence discounted as significant. If nurses fail to recognise their experiences as valuable then why should they bother to reflect and write about them? Understanding this question emphasizes how crucial it is for practitioners who work together to have defined the nature of their work. Also to have made explicit and recognize as valid and valuable their contribution in caring. I feel that, through reflection, the nurse can learn to value these aspects of her work.

Besides sharing experiences using the model of structured reflection, the practitioner may need to share experiences that are of more immediate concern. In my experience this always becomes an opportunity for the supervisor to confront the practitioner to explore more appropriate ways of dealing with stress rather than using supervision as an opportunity to offload anxiety.

Other experiences for reflection can arise from the supervisor prompting the practitioners to confront taken for granted aspects of practice. For example the practitioner may say: 'I gave Mrs Jones her usual bath this morning.' The supervisor may then stop the practitioner and encourage the practitioner to unpick this comment. For example, I might challenge – 'what is usual about this?' – prompting the practitioner to explore her actions in giving Mrs Jones *her usual bath*.

Maintaining a structured reflective diary

This involves keeping a diary in which to write down reflections on experience, which may then be shared in supervision. Practitioners have

(1) Use an A4 notebook.
(2) Split each page.
(3) Write up diary on left hand side.
(4) Use right hand side for further reflections/analysis notes.
(5) Write up experience same day if possible.
(6) Use actual dialogue wherever possible to capture the situation.
(7) Make a habit of writing up at least one experience per day.
(8) Balance problematic experiences with satisfying experience.
(9) Challenge yourself at least once a day about something that you normally do without thought/take for granted – ask yourself – 'why do I do that?' (i.e. make the normal problematic)
(10) Always endeavour to be open and honest with yourself – find the authentic 'you' to do the writing.

Fig. 8.2 Guided reflection – guidelines for keeping a reflective diary.

often said to me – 'I wish I had written it down' as they struggle to recount exactly what happened. The supervisor helps the practitioner to structure her diary to focus on particular experiences that are emerging as significant for her. (See Fig. 8.2.) Focusing experiences in this way is fundamental to the concept of reflexivity – in that it enables the practitioner to come to see themselves differently over a series of similar experiences, and to understand the factors that limit this potential.

Keeping a structured diary also enables the practitioner to undertake periodic reviews of experience in order to make sense of the learning that has taken place over time. This can be linked with formal 'reflective' performance reviews. Linking reflective practice into formal mechanisms is desirable on two counts. Firstly it becomes an organisational as well as a professional activity and hence it is more likely to be recognized as a worthwhile activity by management. This recognition may lead to support for reflective activities. Secondly, from the practitioner's perspective, reviews enable her to fulfil her professional responsibility to demonstrate that she has strived to be most effective in her actions.

Supervision in action

Consider a practitioner who shares with her supervisor how irritated she feels towards an elderly woman who has Parkinson's disease. She knows this woman cannot help herself but becomes frustrated with her slowness in talking and eating. The practitioner recognizes how guilty she feels for feeling this way. She says she has shared these feelings with colleagues who say 'don't worry about it – we all feel the same way towards her'. This comment makes her feel even worse because she is the primary nurse and it distresses her to think that all the staff are intolerant towards this lady.

The issues are surely obvious:

(1)	Skills in talking to this woman (and others like her).
(2)	Reasons for irritation.
(3)	Knowing herself, and how patients make her feel.
(4)	Getting support for work.
(5)	Helping her colleagues with similar feelings.

The supervisor can unpick these issues and explore ways of dealing with them, to enable the practitioner to focus on similar events over the coming two weeks with this woman, and to consider similar feelings she harbours towards her other patients. The supervisor may further suggest that when the practitioner is next engaged with this woman, she stops to think about the reflective questions – 'How is this woman making me feel now? How am I responding to her? What interventions shall I use now?' In this way the practitioner becomes increasingly sensitive to herself and to her practice and begins to reflect-in-action (Schön, 1987), or in other words to frame the problem and search for appropriate interventions *whilst in the situation*. She comes to better understand how this woman is feeling trapped inside her disabled body. She then shares this experience with the nurse continuing this lady's care, and encourages this colleague to reflect on her own feelings towards this woman.

The practitioner feels better in the practice situation because she can begin to understand and control her experience. Of course, the woman also feels better, because she is no longer being rejected and feels that someone is trying to understand and respond to her needs. In the next supervision session, the practitioner reflects on this experience. She says she feels much better now working with this woman although she still found it difficult to talk with her. The supervisor suggests she spends time exploring with this woman how she feels about having Parkinson's disease and to write about the outcome of this interaction in the patient's notes. The practitioner learns that enabling this woman to share her feelings about being disabled enables her to feel positive towards this lady. She is learning the value of developing relationships with people in order to understand who they are.

The process of supervision

The process of supervision is illustrated with a dialogue taken from a supervision session between myself and Gemma, an associate nurse.

The following extract is taken from Gemma's sixteenth session, 11 months after she commenced work at the hospital as an associate nurse. It is her first post since graduating from university with a degree in nursing. Although the sessions are planned to be held at 14 day intervals it is 20 days since her previous session. The delay was caused by difficulty in arranging a mutually convenient date.

The session lasted for one hour. The dialogue was collected from notes taken by the supervisor during the session. Notes are useful:

(1) To enable the practitioner to validate the content of the session.
(2) To enable continuity of the sessions over time by picking up 'cues' from the previous session's notes.
(3) To provide a record for both supervisor and practitioner to analyse or for reflective review.
(4) To enable the practitioner the opportunity for a further level of reflection in reading the notes.

Gemma – supervision session 16

CJ: 'Are there any issues from the notes?'
GEMMA: 'No'
CJ: 'I noted that I set you a task in our previous session?'
(The task was for Gemma to focus on the impact of her feelings on how she approached patients. This had been recognized as a problem for her to focus on.)
GEMMA: 'Yes, there is a situation related to this – not about a patient but about a relative which I wrote about'
CJ: 'Are we going to talk about that?'
GEMMA: 'Sort of...'
(Gemma described her experience of helping the wife of Barry, a man recently admitted with an acute stroke, to wash him one evening. She used the model of structured reflection to compose this account.
GEMMA: 'I think we all found Barry difficult to care for because he was physically heavy. But his wife was adamant – she wanted him home and to be involved in his care ... the wife, she was quite an abrupt lady ... I don't think she meant it nastily ... just her manner. She kept telling us how much she had cared for people – like Barry – in the past ... but, despite trying to pin her down, she wouldn't say in what capacity.
CJ: 'Was that important to know – "in what capacity"?'
GEMMA: 'I think it would have helped a lot – because we could have established her knowledge base then. When I had heard that she wanted to be so involved I felt a huge respect for her ... because that's how I would want to be if Tim (her husband) was ill ... I felt really positive about the situation – I felt I could be of help...'

CJ: 'I felt I could be of help?'

GEMMA: 'In empowering her to have and to care for Barry at home.'

CJ: 'OK'

GEMMA: 'One evening she asked me to help her wash Barry before she went home ...'

CJ: 'Is that a pattern – that she had taken that aspect of care over?'

GEMMA: 'We washed him in the morning – she came in every afternoon and evening and gave him a wash then'

CJ: 'So she always gave him a wash then?'

GEMMA: 'Yes ... I went along to help her ... I gave her control of the situation ... but when it came to ... when I could see there were places that I could help ... suggesting to her different things to her ... she wouldn't have any of it ... I felt humiliated almost ... I wanted to be of help to her ... she wouldn't acknowledge my experience/skills ...'

CJ: 'You felt rejected?'

GEMMA: 'Definitely ... I felt frustrated as well ... I had so many good intentions in helping with this family ... in a way, in a small way, I felt as though I was almost failing Barry ... if I had been more assertive he could have had things done more comfortably'

CJ: 'Could Barry speak?'

GEMMA: 'If he wanted to ... sometimes it was just nonsense ... I identified further down the model (of SR) how I could have reacted, I've written – "If Barry had been upset he would have said something" – he made his feelings clear to us on several occasions that he didn't want us to do things in a certain way ...'

CJ: 'He was happy with what his wife was doing?'

GEMMA: 'In that situation – yes ... but maybe he didn't know it could have been done more comfortably – it links with what you were saying at the beginning (how our feelings towards patients/relatives affect our availability to them – because after that I felt it very very hard to be available to Mrs Taylor (wife)'

CJ: 'Have you written about how you dealt with it?'

GEMMA: 'I've written about my reaction and how I could have dealt with things differently.'

CJ: 'Do you want to share that?'

GEMMA: 'My reaction was frustration ...'

CJ: 'And dealing with it differently?'

GEMMA: 'To be more assertive with her ... but to phrase my assertiveness differently to her'

CJ: 'Did you think "this is no big deal" and just accept their position?'

GEMMA: 'I noted that as a possibility ... but my feelings were stronger than that and I knew I had to work out something different from that'

CJ: 'Do you think your feelings clouded the issue for you?'

GEMMA: 'I don't think so ... without those feelings I don't think I would have identified the issue ...'

CJ: 'Let me just clarify this experience ... Barry has suffered a stroke. His wife asked you to help her wash him – which she did every evening. You perceived that this could be done in a more comfortable way for Barry. She rejected this help. You took this rejection personally and turned around your positive thoughts towards her. You then felt less available to her?'

GEMMA: 'Yes'

CJ: 'And your strategy is to be more assertive with her?'

GEMMA: 'Yes ... instead of saying to her "How about doing it this way" – to say something like "Can I show you how I would roll Barry"'

CJ: 'How do you feel about this experience now?'

GEMMA: 'I don't feel bad about this situation'

CJ: 'Can you see other options? Have you shared it with the primary nurse?'

GEMMA: 'To some extent'

CJ: 'Is there some "game plan" around counselling and teaching his wife?'

GEMMA: 'There wasn't ... but after that I suggested to Leslie that we should have one (Leslie is the primary nurse)

CJ: 'And did he respond?'

GEMMA: 'No ... not really ... because he was getting even more wound up about this woman ...

CJ: 'Right ... other members of the staff are having similar feelings ... so they were likely to reject her as well?'

GEMMA: 'Uh-hmm'

CJ: 'Another option might be to have used confrontation'

GEMMA 'A sense of *déja vu* (laughs) ...'

CJ: 'Yes ... visions of Mrs Kitchen and Mrs Riley!'

I went on to outline and explore with Gemma various significant issues within this experience, for example using confrontation interventions to challenge Mrs Taylor's restricted beliefs, values, behaviour. I also role modelled how she could give Mrs Taylor feedback of her impact on herself.

We explored getting into win–lose situations with patients, where it becomes a personal issue rather than a therapeutic issue, and then explored Gemma's negative feelings and ways these can be dealt with 'positively' through using cathartic interventions (Heron, 1989), for example saying to Mrs Taylor – 'It must be tough for you to see Barry like this.' We also explored her associate nurse responsibility and her communication patterns with the primary nurse.

A number of points are useful to highlight from this dialogue:

(1)   How issues are picked up from one session to the next which led into Gemma sharing her experience with Mrs Taylor, and then relating it to similar experiences with Mrs Kitchen and Mrs Riley.

(2)   The concept of tasks. These tasks usually involve Gemma in relating practice to any relevant theory or structuring her diary to focus on specific experiences.

(3)   How Gemma surfaces her own values of caring which clearly are used to judge the values of the wife in this situation. It is important that Gemma learns to put her own values into perspective in order not to be judgmental about the wife.

(4)   How I clarify issues as they emerge in the session in order to frame issues. This process gives feedback to Gemma that I am listening and to help her focus the issues for reflection.

(5)   At the end of the session Gemma felt her anger towards Mrs Taylor had dissipated. She felt confident. I believe it is crucial that sessions end positively.

Exercises

Note how Carper's (1978) ways of knowing are apparent within this experience. Make a note of these. In particular consider how the ethics surrounding Gemma's perceived role as advocate for Barry are crucial for Gemma to understand.

Can you identify with Gemma's experience? Reflect on how you dealt with similar experiences to Gemma's. Use the model for structured reflection to guide you.

Conclusion

Through guided reflection the practitioner's sense of awareness, curiosity, reflectiveness, and of commitment can be nurtured. Of course, many practitioners already have these qualities. Guidance helps to make the practitioner become selfconscious of these qualities and to give them purpose and direction towards the goal of effective work.

Clearly it will be helpful to the reflective practitioner if her manager is committed to the same therapeutic values and offers positive encouragement to fulfil her therapeutic potential. Without support the reflective practitioner is likely to become increasingly stressed as she struggles against an unyielding and unsympathetic organisation. Just as therapeutic work can be arduous, so can reflection. They naturally parallel each other. Both can be intimate and distressing at times. However the reward for this commitment is fulfilment of therapeutic potential and the satisfaction that comes from achieving this. My experience in working with reflective practitioners has convinced me that access to this therapeutic potential and the satisfaction it brings is achieved through reflection. Dare we resist it?

References

Belenky, M.F., Clinchy, B.M., Goldberger, N.R. & Tarule, J.M. (1986) *Women's Ways of Knowing.* Basic Books, New York.

Boud, D., Keogh, R. & Walker, D. (1985) Promotion reflection in learning: a model. In Boud, D., Keogh, R., Walker, D. (Eds) *Reflecting: Turning Experience into Learning.* Kogan Page, London.

Brookfield, S.D. (1987) *Developing Critical Thinkers.* Open University Press, Milton Keynes.

Carper, B. (1978) Fundamental ways of knowing in nursing. *Advances in Nursing Science,* **11** 13–23.

Dewey, J. (1933) *How We Think.* D.C. Heath, Boston.

Fay, B. (1987) *Critical Social Science,* Polity Press, Cambridge.

Hawkins, P. & Shohet, R. (1989) *Supervision in the Helping Professions.* Open University Press, Milton Keynes.

Heron, J. (1989) *Six Category Intervention Analysis.* Human Potential Resource Group, University of Surrey, Guildford.

James, N. (1989) Emotional labour. *The Sociological Review,* **37.1**, 15–42.

Johns, C.C. (1992) The Burford Nursing Development Unit holistic model of nursing practice. *Journal of Advanced Nursing,* **16** 1090–8.

Johns, C.C. (1993) Professional supervision. *Journal of Nursing Management,* **1** 9–18.

Jourard, S. (1971) *The Transparent Self.* Van Nostrand, Norwalk, New Jersey.

Lawler, J. (1991) *Behind the Screens.* Churchill Livingstone, Melbourne.

Loganbill, C., Hardy, E. & Delworth, U. (1982) Supervision, a conceptual model. *The Counselling Psychologist,* **10.1** 3–42.

Marshall, J. (1980) Stress amongst nurses. In Cooper, C.L., Marshall, J. (Eds), *White Collar and Professional Stress,* 19–62. John Wiley & Sons, Chichester.

Menzies Lyth, I.P. (1988) The functioning of social systems as a defence against anxiety. In *Containing Anxiety in Institutions,* 43–85. Free Association Books, London.

Mezirow, J. (1981) A critical theory of adult learning and education. *Adult Education,* **32.1** 3–24.

Morse, J.M. (1991) Negotiating commitment and involvement in the nurse–patient relationship. *Journal of Advanced Nursing,* **16** 455–68.

OPDC (undated) Supervision; OPDC, YPDC, Yeovil.

Schön, D.A. (1987) Educating the Reflective Practitioner. Jossey-Bass, San Francisco.

Van Hooft, S. (1988) Caring and professional commitment. *The Australian Journal of Advanced Nursing*, **4.4**, 29–38.

Chapter 9
Exemplars of Reflection: Other People Can Do It, Why Not You Too?

This chapter is included in order to give you a chance to experience how nurses can and do reflect. It should enable you to consider others' efforts at reflection in a way that may motivate you into trying out reflection for yourself. As you may have gathered from other chapters of the book, reflection is not always an easy road to take, and you may even feel disheartened by some of the more articulate examples illustrated here, wondering if you could really be so thoughtful about your own practice in order to grow and learn from it. Rest assured however that every contributor to this chapter had to begin the journey somewhere and each has survived to find that reflection can enhance their ability to learn continually from their experience in practice. You now have the benefit of sharing in their efforts, and it is hoped that they may guide you a little, first of all in deciding to reflect at all as well as suggesting a few frameworks for reflection that may prove useful.

Why bother to reflect at all?

If human beings did not possess the ability to be thoughtful about existence, about the problems of life, one could question whether man would for instance ever have harnessed the benefits of fire, or invented the wheel. Some cynics amongst you may no doubt declare at this point that the trouble with mankind could be that sometimes he thinks too much, and does not develop and learn from this great capacity.

It is at this stage that the ability to reflect rather than just be thoughtful could be said to be worth dwelling on. Jarvis (1992) suggests that reflection is not just thoughtful practice but a learning experience. Just as in life, nursing involves situations that are complex, and if we want to understand what nursing is about, we need to try to make sense of these situations. The trouble with nursing as with life is that it is dynamic, constantly changing, frustrating, challenging, exciting, all at the same time! We cannot capture it in tablets of stone and declare that we have 'nursing in the bag', that we know all there is to know or that we have reached a final understanding of practice.

However what we can resolve to do is explore ourselves, by reflecting on our experiences in order to become more self aware and self evaluative. We must grow and learn instead of just relying on ritualization and automatic pilot to get us through a day's work (Street (1991), Saylor (1990), Schön (1983)). Jarvis (1992) talks about the need for reflection because nurses are dealing with people who because of their individual nature require us to be responsive and reflective, instead of simply carrying out routine, ritual and presumption.

In order to be effective we need to be purposeful and goal-directed (Street, 1991), thus reflection is not just about understanding but it is also about changing practice. It is possible to foresee a time in the future, perhaps when theory development could arise from practice, because of a move toward a more reflective way of practising nursing, giving nurses the insight to grow nursing theory from practice itself.

A word of caution is justified at this point. It may be that reflection could offer us a route toward exploring our ability to be therapeutic in our practice by fostering self awareness and an ability to be constructively critical. It may even offer us ammunition in the fight for significant changes within the health service today by allowing us to illustrate why quality and not always quantity is important. We may pay a price for this however, although it could be one that is worthwhile in the long run, since reflection may not always be comfortable; this point being amply illustrated through some of the exemplars. It may force us to face incongruity and undesirable facts about nursing and the health service as a whole, thus one must consider both the positive and negative aspects before embarking on a reflective pathway.

In summary throughout the chapter you should be able to identify the concepts just described, illustrated in the exemplars given. That is to say:

(1) The view that situations in nursing can be complex.
(2) The resolve to try to understand what nursing is about.
(3) The striving to be self aware and to self evaluate.
(4) The questioning of routinization/ritualization.
(5) The efforts to change and challenge current practice.

Helping you to start

The following hints may be worth considering:

Using a framework to help you reflect

Four references to frameworks are given starting on page 134. They are illustrative of the type of tools that qualified and unqualified nurses have used to date, in order to help them with their reflection.

Finding a colleague/mentor/supervisor with whom to reflect

S/he can provide a sounding board, open up different perspectives and provide support and guidance. A relationship built on trust is required however, if the reflective practitioner is to share and explore with another. The role of mentor is explored in more depth in Chapter 3, similarly Chapter 8 explores individual supervision. You may find it useful to reread these chapters, when deciding on setting up a relationship with a mentor or supervisor.

Keeping a reflective journal or diary

Keeping a diary is an extremely useful tip; since memory of events can fade quickly even amongst those of us with the most photographic of memories. It is worth setting aside time to write in your diary, in whatever form feels comfortable to you. It may also be worth choosing an attractively bound file or book in which to record your reflections, as the aesthetics of this do encourage some people to write. In Chapter 8, there are some clear guidelines on how to manage a reflective diary which you may or may not find comfortable to use for yourself.

You may wish to record experiences concerning your own patients or situations that seemed dramatic or special in practice. However it is possible to miss out seemingly routine or mediocre events which on reflection could prove to be useful learning experiences. (See the exemplar on giving an injection for instance.) Of course human nature being what it is, diary keeping requires motivation and commitment. From experience some people do find it easier than others. The most important thing however is to find a method that works well for you.

Reading the literature

Obviously we hope this book will prove useful in providing you with some background on reflection. It is sensible to ensure that you understand the concepts involved and have a clear idea of what you personally find helpful. Chapter 5, which explores the underlying theory behind reflection may prove useful.

Having the courage to change and/or challenge

As mentioned previously reflection can be painful as well as enlightening, bringing things to conscious thought that need to be dealt with, if we wish to live with ourselves as professional practitioners. This is not easy and may be a good reason to find a good mentor/supervisor and exercise careful thought before one embarks on the process. Of course it is helpful if one works in an atmosphere where change and constructive challenge are inherent in the workplace, and thus it is easier then to be brave. If you are not in such a position it is well worth seeking out supportive and facilitative networks, before setting off on the reflective pathway.

A framework for reflection

For someone filled with enthusiasm to begin reflection, the dilemma of 'where do I start?' can spring to mind rapidly. It seems helpful therefore to include several suggestions to use as a framework for going about the business of reflection. It may be that you feel comfortable with one particular framework and opt to use it, every time you reflect. This does not mean that a framework is essential, indeed in my experience, some practitioners do not use one at all. The suggestions here are not the only means available; there are more available in the literature e.g. Mezirow (1981), Burnard (1991), Boud, Keogh & Walker (1985) all provide examples, and no doubt more will emerge as reflection develops in nursing. I include the examples given below because they are ones that I know practitioners have used and found successful:

The reflective cycle

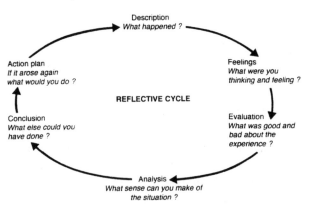

Fig. 9.1   The reflective cycle (from Gibbs, 1988).

Since reflection is not a static process, but one which is dynamic, it seems appropriate to utilise a cyclical approach to it. The reflective cycle illustrated here is adapted from a framework for experiential learning and guides the user through a series of questions, in order to provide structure for an experience reflected on. The reflective practitioner begins initially at the top of the cycle, asking the question – what happened? and then progresses around the cycle in order to explore an experience in practice and guide the reflective process.

Model for structured reflection

This framework and its use in practice are described in detail in Chapter 8 on Guided Reflection and supervision. It is composed of a series of questions helping the reflective practitioner to tune into an experience, and provide structure as above.

Goodman's levels of reflection

Goodman (1984) distinguishes three levels of reflection which the reflective practitioner may achieve. Again these levels could serve as a

---

1st level
Reflection to reach given objectives: Criteria for reflection are limited to technocratic issues of efficiency, effectiveness and accountability.

2nd level
Reflection on the relationship between principles and practice: There is an assessment of the implications and consequences of actions and beliefs as well as the underlying rationale for practice.

3rd level
Reflection which besides the above incorporates ethical and political concerns: Issues of justice and emancipation enter deliberations over the value of professional goals and practice and the practitioner makes links between the setting of everyday practice and broader social structure and forces.

Fig. 9.2 Levels of reflection (Goodman, 1984).

framework, for the practitioner to assess where their quality and depth of reflection lies. Goodman's work in fact forms the basis of the grading criteria upon which undergraduate students' learning contracts are assessed at Oxford Brookes University. This is discussed in more detail in Chapter 2.

Core question – What information do I need access to in order to learn through this experience?

Cue questions –

1.0 *Description of experience*
 .1 *Phenomenon* – Describe the 'here and now' experience.
 .2 *Causal* – What essential factors contributed to this experience?
 .3 *Context* – What are the significant background actors to this experience?
 .4 *Clarifying* – What are the key processes (for reflection) in this experience?

2.0 *Reflection*
 .1 What was I trying to achieve?
 .2 Why did I intervene as I did?
 .3 What were the consequences of my actions for:
 – Myself?
 – The patient/family?
 – For the people I work with?
 .4 How did I feel about this experience when it was happening?
 .5 How did the patient feel about it?
 .6 How do I know how the patient felt about it?

3.0 *Influencing factors*
 .1 What internal factors influenced my decision making?
 .2 What external factors influenced my decision making?
 .3 What sources of knowledge did/should have influenced my decision making?

4.0 Could I have dealt better with the situation?
 .1 What other choices did I have?
 .2 What would be the consequences of these choices?

5.0 *Learning*
 .1 How do I *now* feel about this experience?
 .2 How have I made sense of this experience in light of past experiences and future practice?
 .3 How has this experience changed my ways of knowing:
 – empirics?
 – aesthetics?
 – ethics?
 – personal?

Fig. 9.3 Model of structured reflection (Johns (1992) and Carper (1978)).

A student's own framework for reflection

Finally I have chosen the framework outlined in Chapter 4. Again it poses a series of questions for the practitioner to work through when reflecting on a practice experience. It has emerged from the experiences of a student nurse immersed in reflection over the past four years, and it has obviously worked well for her as a framework to guide a reflective thinking process.

Choose a situation on your placement

Ask yourself...

- What was my role in this situation?
- Did I feel comfortable or uncomfortable? Why?
- What actions did I take?
- How did I and others act?
- Was it appropriate?

- How could I have improved the situation for myself, the patient, my mentor?
- What can I change in future?
- Do I feel as if I have learnt anything new about myself?

- Did I expect anything different to happen?
  What and why?
- Has it changed my way of thinking in any way?
- What knowledge from theory and research can I apply to this situation?
- What broader issues, for example ethical, political or social, arise from this situation?
- What do I think about these broader issues?

Stephenson (1993)

Exemplars from practice

The following examples of reflection are contributed by nurses both qualified and unqualified, who work in Oxfordshire Health Authority. These examples are presented as written by these nurses and have not been altered in any way by the editor. They simply serve to illustrate nurses reflecting on their practice.

There are six excerpts in all, as identified below:

(1) A second year degree student reflecting on and describing caring for an elderly patient with sensory difficulties.
(2) A second year degree student working in a community hospital reflecting on communication and dying.
(3) A third year degree student working on a medical ward, reflecting on the basic tasks of physical caring.
(4) A third year degree student working on a surgical ward, reflecting on support for a patient who had received bad news.
(5) A staff nurse working with a student nurse facilitating her to give an injection. This example illustrates the staff nurse reflecting on her teaching and the concept of a 'basic routine'.
(6) A staff nurse caring for a primary patient, reflecting on the issues of partnership and advocacy.

Using the exemplars to help you think about reflection

General questions that may be useful in your
consideration of each exemplar

- What levels of reflection is the nurse working through?
- Can you identify points on the reflective cycle that the nurse is working through?
- How much of this excerpt is reflection and how much is description?
- How much does referral back to theory/literature/research help the quality of the nurse's reflection?

Above are a list of general questions that would be useful to refer to as you read each exemplar. Throughout the text however you will find specific question posed, which you should try and think about as you read through an exemplar. The aim being that these should enable you to tune into reflection, hopefully in order to help you with your own initial attempts to start writing.

Exemplar 1

Reflection by a second year degree student working in a community mental health field hospital taken from her learning contract, and used to assess her practical abilities in the placement.

'An important part of my learning on the ward has been taking care of the daily needs of one client. She is partially sighted (can see figures, light and dark), has little feeling in her fingers and toes and mild dysphagia. Mentally she is alert; suffers occasionally with confusion; this was especially so when she had a urinary tract infection, and some problems with short term memory.

When I started my placement she needed total care. This meant that she used the commode (beside her bed). At times when she was confused she would believe it was a chair and would call out that she really needed to go to the loo and became quite distressed. It would take a lot of reassurance and persuasion before she would use it.'

Is there any reflective process in the above?

'She is now able to use the frame and walk to the toilet. She needs to have someone with her as she bumps into things and is still unsteady when mobilizing. She becomes quite angry when being directed when she is using her frame. She says she hates being told what to do. I asked her why she thought we gave directions, she replied 'because you think I'm stupid'. I explained that we were doing it to make her feel safe, she said that she still felt dumb and stupid. It is a very difficult situation because she is very wayward with her frame and did need a lot of input, however input made her angry. The more angry she gets, the more she crashes into things as she tries to move too fast. She is not by any means "stupid", but I appreciate that for someone who wishes to be independent, people telling you what to do must be very frustrating. I try not to be overprotective when walking with her and give her as much space, however if she falls whilst in my care I would be accountable.'

Where does reflection begin in this section and at what level? (see Goodman (1984))

This is an experience seen through the eyes of a second year student, trying to unravel the intricacies of caring for an elderly client with sensory difficulties. It says something to me about the novice level she is at, in trying to piece together the realities of actually physically caring for an elderly person. She extracts specifically the difficulties with the lady's mobility, and it seems to illustrate clearly that she has learnt that good nursing is not just about physically providing resources for a patient but also considering the psychological importance of dependence and lack of former abilities.

Questions

(1) How much of this account is description and how much is reflection?
(2) What new knowledge do you think the student came away with, after describing and reflecting on this incident?
(3) Do you see areas that the student could have explored more, to help her understand the situation more fully?

Exemplar 2

These excerpts are taken from the learning contract of a second year degree student on placement in a community hospital

'I was very much looking forward to working at the community hospital as I had heard that there were plenty of opportunities to give 'hands-on' care. I was looking forward to being able to make someone's stay in hospital a pleasant one – by building up a good interpersonal relationship and letting them know that I cared and that I was there for them.

The only thing which worried me about working on a ward with elderly patients, was that I did not want to see anyone die. On my previous ward, one of my patients was extremely ill and it was thought that she was going to die. She did not die, but the days I experienced caring for her when she was so ill, shook me up a great deal. I suddenly realized that we are going to die at some time and that no one can escape. I found this realization hard, as I could not (and still cannot) come to terms with the fact that I am going to die. I have so much to live for and find the prospect of dying quite horrific. I want to live until I've done all the things I've wanted to do – and at the moment, there are so many things I want to accomplish, that it seems I will have to live for a few hundred years!'

At what level is the student reflecting here? (i.e. Goodman (1984)).

'Because of these feelings, I did not want to see anyone die, as this would bring the realization closer. I talked to my mentor about this, and she thought that if anyone should die while I was on the ward, it would be beneficial for me to help lay the body out as I would then confront my feelings and not build any more barriers up, about this.

Thinking about my main fear as to why I don't want to die, it is because there are many things I want to accomplish. Elderly people may have accomplished everything (or nearly everything) that they set out to do. Therefore, why should I find it sad if they die? Perhaps they want to die? I have thought about this a great deal and realized that it is sometimes only sad for the people left behind when an elderly person dies.

Lucy (the patient with the burns on her right leg) told me that since her husband's death, all she wanted to do was to die. I suppose this is a natural feeling as her companion (her life) had been taken away from her and she probably felt that there was nothing left for her on earth. Thus, should it be regarded as sad, that she wants to die, so that she can be with her husband again?

As I said earlier, it is sad when someone dies, as it is so final. Perhaps a relative feels that he/she did not express how he/she really felt to the person, before he/she died. Thus, the relative might feel guilty, lonely and desperately sad. If though, a person strongly believes in God and heaven, then the prospect of dying might not be so frightening. If a person is very religious, then going to heaven can only be a good thing. After all, heaven is meant to be a much nicer place than earth and it is a "place" where you can once again meet up with lost relatives.

What I think I have concluded from all of this, is that feelings about death and dying are very personal. How someone feels about this, is influenced by their religious beliefs, and by their life's experiences. I think we must remember how we feel towards death and dying, when we deal with our patients. There may be many conflicting ideas going through their minds as well. Also, if someone dies in a four bedded bay, how do the other three patients feel? The death of a patient may not only stir the thoughts of the nurses. How does it influence the patients?'

Can you see any evidence of a cyclical process of reflection occurring?

'Overall, an elderly person often feels like a teenager inside an old body. This must be considered when dealing with an elderly person. Also, the patient's thoughts towards growing older, death and dying have to be considered – someone might be feeling as scared and apprehensive as I am.'

Can you identify any assumptions made by the student?

'On the other hand, an elderly patient may feel ready to die – and no longer wants to fight on. This too, has to be considered and respected.'

Again, this is work produced by a second year undergraduate student. It appears to me to show much greater reflection than the last exemplar. Perhaps this is due to the calibre of the student or the fact that it is easier to reflect more profoundly on such a dramatic issue as death and dying? I feel it does demonstrate a process of developing thinking by the student and alludes to the ability of her mentor to offer support in working through some of her fears.

Exemplar 3

This is the reflection of a third year degree student working on a medical ward, on the basic tasks of physical caring

> 'Emphasis on the psychosocial aspects of care can be seen as a praiseworthy attempt to redress the perceived imbalance of an excessively physical orientation on the part of nurses ... (however) nursing remains embroiled in physical care which involves contact with the mess and dirt of bodily life, even while it is aspiring to the "cleaner" caring that deals with people's minds and emotions'.

> Dunlop (1986)

> 'In an analysis of the ward as a learning environment Fretwell (1980) concludes that students frequently perceive the performance of "basic tasks" (that is, those which are commonplace, repetitive and predominantly physical) as routine and presenting few opportunities to enhance professional knowledge and competence. Drawing upon Field's (1981) example "A Phenomenological Look at Giving an Injection" the following excerpts examine in detail two ostensibly "basic physical tasks": feeding and bathing. Paterson and Zderad (1976) have argued that nursing "holds the possibility for both persons to effect and be affected". The intention is therefore to explore

> • How this act is (apparently) experienced by that patient.
> • The impact of this act upon the nurse–patient relationship.
> • How this act is experienced by the nurse.'

Only feeding is included in this exemplar.

Feeding I
'This particularly frail and emaciated 86 year old gentleman presented with digoxin toxicity. He also suffered from progressive cardiac failure, osteoarthritis and bilateral cataracts.

Observing this gentleman's unsuccessful attempts to manipulate cutlery and manoeuvre food to his mouth before finally pushing aside the uneaten meal was a sobering lesson. Had I inadvertently contributed, albeit in a minor and unobtrusive manner, to the endemic of hospital-induced malnutrition? Although conscientiously providing a high density diet to compensate for his meagre appetite, enthusiastically encouraging him to eat small quantities frequently and arranging every conceivable need within his grasp, I had, nonetheless, neglected the simple mechanics of the process. To his arthritic hands a sealed dessert represented an impenetrable barrier: an additional and unnecessary frustration for him and food for thought indeed.'

At what point on the reflective cycle would you identify the above?

'The most obvious solution also seemed the least desirable. Would feeding this gentleman preserve his fragile self-esteem or be interpreted as a humiliating and undignifying insult, a further and unwelcome confirmation of his increasing disability? Was it necessary to compromise his sensibilities in order to ensure he ate enough?'

Can you identify with the above dilemma?

'Planning with him an acceptable diet revealed additional problems. The size of meals posed an uninviting ordeal sufficient to dampen his appetite. An impaired ability to smell, taste and see food deprived him of the stimulus to eat; pain and hunger were experienced as similar and frequently confused sensations. Although equipped with complete dentures chewing was both arduous and exhausting. The three meal-a-day hospital regimen was dissimilar from his accustomed habit. The embarrassment of constipation and of faecal incontinence was incentive enough to avoid eating.

I endeavoured to forewarn him of an impending meal and, prior to its arrival, encouraged him to visualize its contents in an attempt to whet his appetite; a mint aperitif refreshed his mouth and stimulated gastric motility. I adjusted his position, tucked a napkin onto his chest and arranged his food in a clock-face to assist him locate each mouthful. Broad-handled utensils and gentle coaxing compensated for his loss of dexterity. A small, semi-liquid and strong-flavoured meal, supplemented by between-meal snacks (Buildup), proved more palatable and manageable. Replenishing a beaker of fruit juice and inviting him to use a drinking-straw provided readily accessible fluid.'

Has the student's thinking moved on through the reflective cycle to a different point?

'Sharing and resolving the eating problems encountered by this gentleman demonstrated, I believe, a genuine concern for his well-being and contributed in some small degree toward rejuvenating his diminished sense of personal effectiveness and self worth.'

'... the lack of consciousness of the other separates him from his environment, creating a barrier to his interaction with external things ... He lies before me an uncommunicating being. It is easy to deny him the right of existence, to objectify his presence and deny that he experiences sensory feelings'

Field (1981)

Can you identify a process of learning and analysis that would influence the way this student dealt with a similar situation, in the future?

Feeding II

'This 42 year old lady had suffered diffuse cerebral lesions secondary to bacterial meningitis and an episode of cardio-respiratory failure. Although presently in a stable condition her prognosis remained uncertain. Her level of conscious responsiveness was greatly reduced. She received a pump-delivered elemental diet via nasogastric intubation.

I was denying her choice, dictating when she took food and drink, how often and in what combination. A tasteless, untextured and precisely balanced meal devoid of the enjoyment with which I associate food: merely a means of subsistence. How will I know if she is satisfied? Does she experience hunger or thirst? Is the tube an unpleasant sensation and how might I alleviate this discomfort? How can I minimize the risk of her vomiting and ensure the tube is correctly located?

Her body, once a private domain, has been relegated to a collective concern: she had surrendered her most intimate social space to the intrusive vagaries of those upon whom she depends. I fail to obtain gastric aspirate but receive satisfactory sounds from a generous injection of air. I explain the rationale for this procedure and apologize for the discomfort I imagine it has inflicted.

As Naisbitt (1984) predicted, with these technological innovations there seems to be a proportionate need on the part of individuals for more touch – the reassurance and security communicated by the presence of another person. I gently massage her hands.'

The student nurse, in a similar way to one of the staff nurse exemplars, is reflecting on what initially seems part of basic routine or everyday nursing care. It demonstrates the strength of not simply relying on reflection to analyse dramatic events in one's nursing, but to utilise the process to examine everyday issues and thus try to learn from them. Quite simply it identifies a sensitivity and humility, which allows the student to reflect on the lived experience of his patients, which can so easily be taken for granted.

Exemplar 4

A third year degree student working on a surgical ward reflects on supporting a patient who has received bad news.

'Jean had been admitted to the ward for investigations into slight liver pain. She had a history of cancer of the bowel – which had been surgically removed and was understandably anxious about her diagnosis this time. From the previous day's investigations she had been told that they had found a tumour in her liver and that surgery may be needed. Further tests were needed to determine the size and extent of the tumour. When I met Jean she was very cheerful but a little anxious about having the tests – I think she was more worried about undergoing these tests than the actual results. We built up an instant rapport and I was able to spend a lot of time with her explaining what was going to happen and actually accompany her down to X-ray for angiograms. During the angios I found it hard to see anything on the X-rays and the radiologist did not seem to want to point anything out to me.

After returning to the ward, Jean seemed relaxed and glad that the tests were over. I was with her when the ward round reached her and the surgeon explained to her that she had an inoperable liver tumour and that there was nothing more he could do for her. Whilst delivering his bad news he sat beside her and held her hand – and offered help with any questions she had – however as soon as he had finished he left quickly. His houseman stood at the bottom of the bed throughout all this, David, the co-ordinator (staff nurse), was present and I was sat in a chair beside her bed. At the time, she was very shocked and seemed concerned about further tests – she was reassured by the surgeon that tests were no longer needed and that surgery was pointless. As soon as everyone else left – Jean completely broke down, she was completely shocked and stunned and all I could do was to hold her hand and let her cry.'

Is the above description or reflection?

'I felt extremely upset by this news and found it very difficult not to just cry with her. Although I have nursed dying patients, Jean did not seem the same as these. She was healthy, had a large happy family and enjoyed life – I felt I saw her as a person and not just as a patient and identified with her personality. I experienced a great deal of empathy for her and felt completely useless and desperate to comfort her. I've never been in that situation before and just did not feel that anything I could say would help. I felt a huge deficit in my ability to comfort her and we just sat in silence – squeezing each other's hands, Jean weeping and me close to tears. I went to make her a cup of tea and the other team members offered support and offered to take over for me – but I wanted to stay with her. I felt I owed it to her, I did not feel ashamed of how upset I was, as I felt this was perfectly natural, Jane (staff nurse) came over and supported me with Jean at first, but I soon realized that there are no correct words or ways to deal with these situations and that our time and understanding are the only things we can give at that moment, and Jean did feel some small comfort just to have me there with her. We talked about her family, her son's wedding and how, now she would be able to attend as she would not be having surgery. She even started to think about the future – saying that she was going to go on holiday now and enjoy life from now onwards.'

Can you identify how the student is reflecting on her initial thoughts and feelings here? How are they helping her to make sense of the situation?

'Although I am familiar with the stages of loss, I feel a great deal of Jean's initial reaction was relief that she would not have to undergo major surgery.

She had expressed huge fears about this previously and I think that she did not fully comprehend what the news actually meant for her future. Indeed, the surgeon did not give her an amount of time that she may have and she did not ask. However, I realise that she had been preparing herself for this and the tension overwhelmed her at the last moment. I strongly believe however, that the doctors could have prepared her and also the nursing staff, a little better, before telling her the prognosis. I understand that the surgeons are busy and cannot lie to their patients during ward rounds but feel that the situation could have been handled more sensitively, e.g. by waiting until he had finished the round and had time to spend with her. Also by limiting the number of staff around at the time and possibly waiting until she had some member of family present for support.'

Can you identify what stage of the reflective cycle (Gibbs, 1988) the student is on?

'I do not know whether I would have handled the situation better if I had been warned, but I would have had time to prepare myself adequately and possibly seek support from trained members of staff. I feel I had such a strong reaction to Jean's case, as my family have been going through similar experiences. My father has recently had surgery for skin cancer and whilst waiting for results – we all experienced feelings of potential loss and grief. I observed my father go through all the phases from denial to acceptance and back to depression and denial again and felt utterly helpless at that time also.'

The student is applying theory to her experiences, although she does not specifically mention her sources. See Kubler-Ross (1970).

'It was extremely frightening to watch my father trying to deal with potential bad news and adapt to the idea that his prognosis may not be promising. This is something that I previously reserved for my professional life not my personal life and found myself completely denying that it was actually my father it was happening to. Jean was concerned for her family and did not want to tell her children (who were all adult). I was able to rely on my own personal experience here as my family took huge comfort from being together and working through our worries and told Jean that her children would want to help her through this and she could find great strength from them, as my father did.

Somehow I had attached all my anxiety onto Jean as I was unable to be present when my father was told his diagnosis and I feel this had a great relevance to my need to help Jean through this time. Although my father has made a full recovery now, the memory of the fears that haunted me whilst waiting for his prognosis helped me to understand a little better how Jean might have felt – although I cannot begin to imagine how I would feel if I was told that I was terminally ill.'

This example illustrates for me, the student going through a discovery of self, as well as showing clearly that applying theory about loss or breaking bad news is not easy in practice. The real learning for this student seems to me to come from her ability to confront the stark reality of dealing with situations such as the above and living through them with the patient. It also demonstrates, I feel, the willingness of this particular student to share some of her own personal and private life experiences as she reflects on the situation. This will inevitably not feel comfortable for some people, especially if one is expected to share reflection with a mentor or supervisor. I would say the choice of how much one wishes to expose or explore must lie with the practitioner themselves.

Exemplar 5

In this exemplar a staff nurse is working with a student nurse facilitating her to give an injection. The example illustrates the staff nurse reflecting on her teaching and the concept of a 'basic routine'.

'*Description*

On a busy morning shift one of the patients expressed that he was in pain post-operatively following a hernia repair. He also felt nauseated and therefore I decided to give him a narcotic and an anti-emetic via an intra-muscular injection, with a view to relieving his symptoms.

I approached the student and asked her if she would help me to check and draw up the injections. She agreed to do this and whilst undertaking the act of "drawing up", I asked her if she had given an injection before. She replied she had given a few but did not elaborate. I then asked her if she would like to give this particular injection. She appeared to hesitate, looked slightly unenthusiastic and said "yes". She then asked me what needle she should use. A short discussion followed on the issue of using blue or green needles for intra-muscular injections, before she decided to use the blue needle. As we approached the patient I suggested she give the two injections together (i.e. via same needle).

Once we had reassured the patient and he was prepared to receive the injection the student set about giving them. Again I suggested she gave them together. The learner then placed the needle into the central part of the patient's buttock and after injecting the contents, removed the syringe and needle, before beginning to proceed to give the second injection. At this point, I suggested she stop and consider the proximity of the sciatic nerve to the penetration of the needle. On hearing this, she looked completely confused and unable to comprehend. I finally pointed to the upper outer quadrant and the student then successfully gave the second injection.'

Notice here how the practitioner has divided description from reflection. It is easy to write merely descriptively, if one has not identified clearly the difference between description and reflection.

'*Reflection*

On looking back at this situation, my feelings go out to the student, as this was not much of a learning experience for her, but a great learning experience for me!

On this particular morning I was under pressure, caring for a number of patients, some of whom had received surgery or were about to go to theatre. Subsequently I was feeling guilty that I was unable to give the student the time she deserved and needed. The student was also being mentored by another member of staff, I did not know her and had not worked with her before. The environment could not be considered satisfactory as both learner and facilitator were under pressure, patient demands were high, the ward was generally busy and noisy, and the patient concerned needed immediate pain relief. The student had said she had given injections in the past. During the time prior to giving the injection she was able to draw up the medications satisfactorily. On these observations I assumed she would need little help and assistance in giving the injection. What did concern me at the time was the apparent lack of motivation and interest in the student's response, when it was suggested that she could give the injection. I put it down to the fact that in already having given injections in the past, she found the experience unchallenging by this stage in her training. In my experience to date, this would certainly seem the case, having given hundreds of injections, to the point of being able to give them in my sleep!'

Think of the basic 'routines' you do on a daily basis and apply one of the reflective frameworks to your thoughts. What issues arise from you doing this?

'Further as practice becomes more repetitive and routine and as knowing-in-practice becomes extremely tacit and spontaneous, the practitioner may miss important opportunities to think about what he is doing.'

Schön (1983)

'Was it possible that I had 'over-learned' (Schön, 1983) this procedure to the extent that I automatically assumed that the student must have also become over familiar with the process of giving an injection? It would seem so.'

Notice how the practitioner has researched the literature to help her to reflect on the difficulties of this situation.

'Once assuming the reason for her lack of enthusiasm, which was later found to be incorrect, I did not stop to consider the other possibilities. Certainly my attitude did not help and I feel this was particularly hindered by the obvious "flimsy" relationship between myself and the student. By not knowing her at all well, communication was not forthcoming.'

Where is the practitioner at now on the reflective cycle' (Gibbs, 1988)?

'That one of the most important of these conditions is the attitudinal quality of the interpersonal relationship between facilitator and learner'

Rogers (1988)

'In having no knowledge of her background of experiences which I would hopefully have gathered previously after her initial arrival to the ward, if I were to be her mentor, I was aware there were gaps needing to be filled. Unfortunately this was not a good or appropriate time to fill them.

Rogers (1988) also states that teachers need to relate as persons to their students. In this case the uniform, job title and the fact that the student did not know me, may have assisted the student in regarding me in the light of a stranger and not as a teacher and facilitator. In order to become a facilitator, Rogers (1988) states one must promote interest, curiosity, initiate questioning and enquiry and provide resources for learning. It is apparent I was having trouble fulfilling the role. The student did question the use of needle which did prompt a short discussion and it made me think about my own practice, temporarily breaking me out of the routine of giving an injection. Giving the injection incorrectly and putting the patient at risk brought it home to me that this experience was not going well, and I now suddenly saw that my lack of preparation was becoming evident.'

'Much reflection-in-action hinges on the experience of surprise. When intuitive spontaneous performance yields nothing more than the results expected from it, then we tend not to think about it.'

Schön (1983) p 56

'Not only had I assumed incorrectly that the student knew how to give an injection, I had assumed she had understood my verbal communication in "giving them together". She had not asked for help in locating the correct area of the buttock, but then I had not encouraged her or questioned her knowledge.'

'Critical thinking and judgment are fostered in an atmosphere where the student can question and dissent without feeling guilty or disloyal.'

Quinn (1988)

'Quinn (1988) goes on to cite Reilly and Oermann (1985) who suggest that teachers may set unrealistic demands on students by expecting them to do everything perfectly.

The importance of making oneself understood is paramount. Again, I assume she understood me and since she did not question my instructions but interpreted that she should give them at the same time, (not together through the same needle) she went ahead with that action. I felt upset that she had misinterpreted my instructions but the fact was, the actual mechanics of giving the injection was correct, and she did not need further instruction in that respect. The patient throughout appeared unaware of what was happening and satisfied that he had received the analgesia and anti-emetic.

What is most unfortunate about this experience is that the student and I did not reflect on her or my actions. The opportunity to discuss the situation did not arise and this gave me feelings of dissatisfaction and inadequacy. At the time I did make a point of praising her practical ability in actually giving the injection.'

'Teachers and students should work together to examine the reasons for failures so as to learn by such mistakes.'

Quinn (1988)

'What is clear is that I have learnt something from this and next time will make adequate preparation beforehand wherever possible. Effort should be made to encourage a better environment to learn in, more time allowed for discussion and gathering of knowledge already gained. Ascertaining the student's particular and personal needs using open questioning is vital. Ensuring time has been allowed to get to know one another as people, preferably away from the clinical environment. In building up a good relationship communication will be more forthcoming and hopefully more clearly understood.'

Can you identify where the practitioner is now on the reflective cycle?

'If necessary it may have been useful to encourage the student to practise injection giving into an orange or piece of foam beforehand and ensure that he or she is aware of the anatomy and physiology of the nervous system in relation to the lower part of the body. This may help promote curiosity and motivation though Carl Rogers (1969) as cited by McMahon & Pearson (1991) states that for learning to be effective the drive and impetus must come from the learner herself. The facilitator should question the learner immediately if enthusiasm and motivation are not apparent, and find out the reasons why. The emphasis is in the enjoyment of learning and learning occurs when the experience is enjoyable.

Finally I should recognize fully my own experiences are a valuable resource for the learner. Knowles (1978) cited by Vaughan and Pilmoor (1989) recognized the uniqueness of each of us in terms of our experience which in itself is the most valuable resource and which should be available to others.

If nothing else I hope I have learnt to recognize the needs of future learners even when it is not obvious and in doing so, help them to learn by facilitation in an enjoyable and stimulating way, making time for reflection and discussion afterwards. I now realize there is much potential for learning even in the small act of giving an injection.'

What else would you reflect on in this situation? Perhaps: lack of time in a busy clinical learning environment? Setting a few ground rules with a learner you hardly know if you lack time.

This account shows very honest and sensitive reflection on the part of the staff nurse. It highlights for me how one cannot ignore even the simplest, most basic areas of routine practice, when considering the facilitation of effective learning.

If we reflect on this in the light of the principles of adult learning, it is possible that the student could have been more forthcoming about her knowledge and skills but for some reason felt unable to express them. She was a very shy student, who did require a lot of support and constant encouragement through this particular placement. The staff nurse is very critical of herself, yet manages to arrive at some constructive analysis that she will not forget when a similar situation occurs again. Through her reflection one can see clearly a process of analysis and critical thought which has enabled her to learn from what she may initially have written off as an unsatisfactory experience. She also uses literature from educationalists and from reflective theorists to enhance her analysis.

Exemplar 6

Here a staff nurse caring for a primary patient, reflects on the issues of partnership and advocacy.

'When Florrie James was allocated to my nursing team and I decided to become her primary nurse, I was aware that she was a very determined woman. She had, for example already pulled her nasogastric tube out, because it was uncomfortable. On initiating our relationship I attempted to approach her in a spirit of partnership though making explicit what my boundaries were. For example she was restricted to 30 ml of fluid per hour. She wanted more so I explained the effect this would have. We agreed that I would return hourly to provide the fluid.

This I did, having determined it was important for her to trust me and our relationship grew. Florrie presented medically with an abdominal obstruction which did not resolve. She was treated conservatively by the doctor as her long standing respiratory problems presented a great anaesthetic risk. By acting as her primary nurse and using the principles of the nursing process I was the care planner and provider for Florrie when I was on duty. Over the period of a week the intimate nature of care provision enabled me to know more of Florrie and I became aware of her desire to wait no longer; she wanted surgery. My instinct was to dissuade her, in fact I expressed to her that I felt she could well die. Her determination was unaffected and so I represented her point of view to the surgeons who undertook to operate and actively treat her. Initially her recovery appeared to go well, the underlying cause of the obstruction was adhesions. Both Florrie and I were optimistic.

However her breathing deteriorated and I was instrumental in arguing for her admission to the intensive care unit. This was in accordance with her previously expressed wish of active treatment, by this time she appeared too hypoxic to make decisions. She was ventilated for several days and returned to us, unfortunately she went into respiratory failure again and died.

Through reflection I realized that my initial view of advocacy had been very simplistic, that I knew best (paternalistic). Had Florrie not been so determined my view might have prevailed, in reality a form of utilitarianism (best for us and her family.). The intimate nature of nursing enhanced by the system of care delivery on the ward (primary nursing) enabled me to know Florrie better and to take the risk of telling her my view (the information was biased!). However in doing so I risked destroying her hope, a risk I would be very careful of taking again. In the context of our relationship it was symptomatic of the honesty that existed; I did not regard myself as a limitless provider as exemplified by my statement of boundaries.'

Can you extract specific issues that the nurse has reflected upon in relation to advocacy?

'The honesty was frightening as it enabled me to realize that I didn't like her very much. I realized that it was probably because she did not flatter me as a nurse or offer me easy options. Once I became aware of this, I was able to progress and offer something deeper. That she always asked for me by name and gave me a kiss on the night before she died were precious rewards.'

Can you identify reflection here that may prove painful for the nurse involved? Does this initiate any moral/ethical dilemmas for the potential reflective practitioner?

'Whilst it would seem to have been appropriate as her primary nurse that I should develop such a closeness the context that I can only be on duty for five out of 15 shifts per week is one to consider. This is where teamwork is essential (we have a structure where there are three teams from which the primary nurses operate). I soon realized that there was a danger of her becoming an 'unpopular patient' (Stockwell, 1972) as she was very demanding of nursing time and energy. So whilst I was able to work with her I needed to be able to give my team the input to sustain such an approach and our morale. That I perhaps did not was contextual to the short time I had been in post and the way in which I felt solely responsible, not necessarily a virtue in a team setting.

When undertaking to represent what she wanted it was a professional concept that motivated me, I had negotiated a partnership and this was the price, for I felt deep personal sorrow and conflict in doing so. It was only just before her death that I began to reconcile the professional versus personal conflict (Gadow, 1980) and moved towards a "fellow feeling" in which my emotions were intense but the form and direction were truly focused on Florrie.

I learnt that to take on the role of an advocate is not always easy and that the examination of my ethical standpoint enlightened me considerably. Such a role may be possible but with its demands not one which can be undertaken with every patient; for example no other patient in my team had such input at the time I was nurse to Florrie.

This apparent difficulty may be because advocacy is being attempted in a system which offers at best "benign paternalism" (Porter, 1988). Indeed it has been argued that it is immoral to instil an awareness of ethical decisions in situations which may prevent their fulfilment (Davis, 1986). My awareness was heightened through my previous learning opportunities (ones only recently being offered to nurses) and my feeling is that whilst I am now able to be more creative in my approach the sense of failure can be stronger. In order to preserve my inner peace I need awareness of what the contextual as well as the personal limitations are. Also that these aspects may be completely outweighed when the positive nature of such endeavours prevails.'

This exemplar appears to me to show a sophisticated level of reflection, that has developed through experience of practice, self awareness and an ability to be self-critical. It also demonstrates how reflective practice can feel uncomfortable, and that one may learn things about one's environment that do not necessarily feel congruent.

Conclusion

In considering these exemplars I have been able to identify a general development in reflective ability as a nurse gains in experience, knowledge and skills. Of course this may not necessarily be the case for every practitioner, since it depends on how one utilizes such experience, knowledge and skills. Also the personal styles of reflective writing are undoubtedly varied, however it appears to me that the use of literature to develop one's thinking is helpful, plus awareness of self is necessary in order to facilitate a depth of reflection.

The exemplars are powerful, particularly in their ability to highlight a process of analytical thinking about practice and a willingness and ability to change and consider practice in relation to it. They also demonstrate that reflection can be painful; however it could be that such an outlet for exploration of emotions is cathartic for the practitioner. Lastly they demonstrate to me that reflection is not just about a way of learning the art and science of nursing, but potentially enables the practitioner to examine and act upon the actual realities of practice, in order to learn from experience.

Now is your chance to try it!

References

Boud, D., Keogh, R. & Walker, D. (1985) (Eds) *Reflection: Turning Experience into Learning.* Kogan Page, London.

Burnard, P. (1991) Improving through reflection. *Journal of District Nursing*, May, 10–12.

Davis, D.S. (1986) Nursing, an ethic of caring. *Human Medicine*, **2**, 20.

Dunlop, M. (1986) Is a science of caring possible? *Journal of Advanced Nursing*, **11**, 661–70.

Field, P. (1981) A phenomenological look at giving an injection. *Advanced Journal of Nursing*, **6**, 291–6.

Fretwell, J. (1980) An enquiry into the ward learning environment. *Nursing Times*, Occ. Paper 76, 16–22.

Gadow, S. (1980) Existential advocacy. Philosophical foundation of nursing. In Spickers, S. & Gadow, S. (Eds) *Nursing Image or Reality*. Springer Publishing Co., New York.

Gibbs, G. (1988) *Learning by Doing. A guide to teaching & learning methods*. Further Education Unit, Oxford Polytechnic, Oxford.

Goodman, J. (1984) Reflection and teacher education: a case study and theoretical analysis. *Interchange*, **15**, 3 9–26.

Jarvis, P. (1992) Reflective practice & nursing. *Nurse Education Today* **12**, 174–1.

Kubler-Ross, E. (1970) *On Death and Dying*, Tavistock, London.

MacMahon, R. & Pearson, A. (1991) *Nursing as Therapy*, Chapman & Hall, London.

Mezirow, J. (1981) A critical theory of adult learning and education. *Adult Education* **32**, 3–24.

Naisbitt, J. (1984) *Megatrends*. Warner Books, New York.

Paterson, J. & Zderad, L. (1976) *Humanistic Nursing*. National League for Nursing, New York.

Porter, S. (1988) Siding with the system. *Nursing Times*, **84**, 41, 30–31.

Quinn, F.M. (1988) *The Principles & Practice of Nurse Education*, 2nd edition. Croom Helm, London & Sydney.

Rogers, C. (1988) *Freedom to learn in the 80s*, Charles E. Merrill Publishing Co, Pyrmont.

Saylor, C.R. (1990) Reflection & professional education: art, science & competency. *Nurse Education*, **15**, No 2, March/April, 8–11.

Schön, D. (1983) *The Reflective Practitioner*. Basic Books, New York.

Stockwell, F. (1972) *The Unpopular Patient*. Royal College of Nursing, London.

Street, A. (1991) *From Image to Action Reflection in Nursing Practice*. Deakin University Press, Geelong.

Vaughan, B. & Pillmoor, M. (1989) *Managing Nursing Work*. Scutari Press, London.

Further reading

Allen, D.G. & Bowers, B. (1989) Willing to learn: a reconceptualization of thinking & writing in the nursing curriculum. *Journal of Nursing Education*, **28**, No 1, 6–11.

Holly, M.L. (1989) Reflective writing and the spirit of inquiry. *Cambridge Journal of Education*, **19**, No 1, 71–80.

Lyte, V.J. & Thompson, J.G. (1990) The diary as a formative teaching and learning aid incorporating means of evaluation and renegotiation of clinical learning objectives. *Nursing Education Today*, **10**, 228–32.

Meerabeau, L. (1992) Tacit nursing knowledge: an untapped resource or a methodological headache? *Journal of Advanced Nursing*, **17**, 108–12.

Powell, J.H. (1989) The reflective practitioner in nursing. *Journal of Advanced Nursing*, **14**, 824–32.

Acknowledgements

My sincere thanks to: Paul Emanual, Kari Lucy, Claudia Mayfield, Julia Mepham, Brigid Reid, and Carol Wells for contributing examples of their work to this chapter.

Index